PCOS FERTILITY BOOK

A Complete Cookbook Diet with More Than 100 Recipes for Women with PCOS to Lose Weight, Boost and Improve Fertility, Reset Hormones, and Fight Against Inflammation with a Natural Insulin Resistant Diet

MIA COLLINS PARKER

© **Copyright 2020 - All rights reserved.**

The content contained within this book may not be reproduced, duplicated or transmitted without direct written permission from the author or the publisher.

Under no circumstances will any blame or legal responsibility be held against the publisher, or author, for any damages, reparation, or monetary loss due to the information contained within this book, either directly or indirectly.

Legal Notice:

This book is copyright protected. It is only for personal use. You cannot amend, distribute, sell, use, quote or paraphrase any part, or the content within this book, without the consent of the author or publisher.

Disclaimer Notice:

Please note the information contained within this document is for educational and entertainment purposes only. All effort has been executed to present accurate, up to date, reliable, complete information. No warranties of any kind are declared or implied. Readers acknowledge that the author is not engaged in the rendering of legal, financial, medical or professional advice. The content within this book has been derived from various sources. Please consult a licensed professional before attempting any techniques outlined in this book.

By reading this document, the reader agrees that under no circumstances is the author responsible for any losses, direct or indirect, that are incurred as a result of the use of the information contained within this document, including, but not limited to, errors, omissions, or inaccuracies.

Table of Contents

Introduction 11
Chapter 1: What You Need to Know About PCOS 14
    Common Signs and Symptoms 15
    What Causes PCOS? 18
    Advice for Newly Diagnosed 20
Chapter 2: Some Tips to Overcome the Common PCOS Symptoms 23
    Tips for Managing Your Emotional and Mental Health .. 23
    Tips for Managing Your Physical Health 27
Chapter 3: The Battle Between PCOS and the Weight Scale 30
    Increment Physical Activity 31
    Follow a Natural and Balanced PCOS Diet 33
Chapter 4: Having PCOS Doesn't Mean You're Infertile 36
    Ovulation in Women 36
    Being Pregnant with PCOS 38
Chapter 5: The Relationship Between PCOS and Chronic Inflammation 40
    Symptoms of Chronic Inflammation 41
    Tips to Control Inflammation 43

Chapter 6: The Link Between PCOS and Insulin Resistance 45
    Symptoms of Insulin Resistance 45
    Understanding the Glycemic Index 47
Chapter 7: Food as a Medicine: A National Balanced and Insulin Resistant Diet 50
    Foods to Consume 50
    Foods to Limit 52
    Foods to Avoid 53
    Tips for a Healthy Diet 54
Chapter 8: Recipes 56
    Breakfast 56
        Kale and Pepper Egg Bake 56
        Microwavable Egg Veggie Breakfast 57
        Navy Bean Egg Scramble 58
        Summer Eggs in a Pan 59
        Egg Casserole with Sweet Potato 61
        Citrus Pineapple Smoothie 62
        Breakfast Smoothie 63
        PB&J Smoothie 64
        Cherry Chocolate and Cinnamon Smoothie 65
        Green Tea Pear Smoothie 66
        Cranberry Quinoa Granola 67

Almond Butter Hot Cereal Instant Flax Meal 68

Nutty Oatmeal with Blueberries 69

Strawberry Breakfast Quinoa 70

Vegetable Hash 71

Almond Pancakes 73

A Simple Low-Carb Breakfast 74

Soup and Salad 76

Tomato Soup 76

Chicken Minestrone 77

Spicy Vegetable Soup 78

Coconut and Ginger Soup 80

Citrus Seafood Soup 82

Turkey and Cauliflower Chowder 83

Split Pea Soup 84

Mediterranean Quinoa Salad 85

Bean and Fruit Salad 88

Coleslaw 89

Thai Tahini Slaw 90

Pecan Spinach Salad 91

Wild Rice Peach Salad 92

Salmon-Arugula Salad 93

Snacks and Sides 94

Zucchini Fries 94

Creamed Spinach and Leeks 95

Spring Vegetable Medley 96

Crispy Onion Rings 97

Spice-Roasted Chickpeas... 99

Sweet Potato Hummus 100

Oat Energy Balls 101

Nutmeg Pear Chips 102

Dill Carrot Ribbons 103

Sweet Potato Salad 104

Bean Cannellini Pilaf... 105

Tomato and Spinach Stuffed Mushrooms................... 106

Roasted Vegetables 108

Brussel Sprouts with Berries and Nuts........................ 109

Vegetarian...110

Crispy Almond Tofu 110

Kale and Tofu Scramble... 112

Grilled Cauliflower Steaks with Black Bean Salsa 113

Split Pea Falafel 115

Cauliflower Fried Rice 116

Southwestern Quinoa Skillet.. 118

Stuffed Mint Eggplant.. 119

Vegetable Pecan Burgers 121

Bean Stuffed Zucchini 122

Mixed Vegetable Lettuce Wraps 124

Southwest Sweet Potatoes 125

Spicy Falafel 126

Farmer's Market Paella 128

Chilled Asian Vegetable Noodles 129

Vegetarian Egg Pizza 130

Southwestern Rice 132

Poultry and Meat 133

Chicken with Ginger Rice Noodles 133

Breaded Chicken with Mustard 135

Chicken and Olives 136

Rosemary Baked Chicken Drumstick 137

Moussaka 138

Chicken Wrap 140

Mediterranean Pork Chops 141

Marinara Meatballs 142

Turkey and Bean Chili 144

Turkey with Peaches and Walnuts 146

Sage Turkey Mix 147

Turkey Burgers with Mango Salsa 148

Pork Fajita Roll-Ups 149

Baked Parsley Lamb.. 150

Fish and Seafood 152

Fish and Orzo 152

Fish Cakes 153

Shrimp and Bean Salad...154

Cod and Mushrooms..156

Creamy Curry Salmon..157

Trout with Tzatziki Sauce 158

Shrimp Mojo de Ajo 159

Five-Spice Calamari 161

Vegetable Baked Salmon 162

Sun-Dried Tomato Cod...163

Honey Salmon 165

Trout with Lemon Sauce... 166

Salmon Wrap 167

Haddock Asian-Style.. 169

Fish Tacos 170

Nut-Breaded Cod with Lemon 172

Salmon with Pistachio Crust 174

Drinks and Dessert 175

Strawberry Lemonade...175

 Iced Green Tea...176

 Green Apple Smoothie..177

 Coconut Custard..178

 Dark Chocolate Chia Pudding 180

 Lemon and Blueberry Curd..181

 Baked Walnut Pears.. 182

Sauce and Dressing... 183

 Spicy Almond Dressing.. 183

 Turmeric Tahini Dressing.. 184

 Smoked Paprika Dressing.. 185

 Sesame Orange Sauce for Stir-Fry 186

 Fiery Peanut Sauce...187

 Tomato Dressing 188

 Easy Marinara Sauce.. 189

Conclusion 191

References 193

Introduction

Once you're diagnosed with PCOS, it's important to understand everything about it, why you have it, and what you can do to ease symptoms. Polycystic Ovary Syndrome (PCOS) receives its name from the numerous small cells, also known as cysts, which appears on your ovaries. They can cause pelvic pain and lead to infertility, as well as cause other health issues. This is one of the reasons, I chose to write this book.

I'm not a doctor and before my diagnosis I've never heard about PCOS. I'm a woman who understands the emotional, mental, and physical challenges of the syndrome. Like you, when I was first diagnosed I was devastated. I didn't know who to turn to, because I wasn't sure if anyone would understand my disease. Over time, I started realizing that I was letting my diagnosis control my life. It's a mistake that lots of women make, but I hope you can quickly and easily overcome your problems by reading my book. It's important to know that PCOS does not control you–you have to control it.

Hopefully, now I'm able to control my body and my mind but this doesn't mean that my feelings still don't creep up. Sometimes my emotions still get the best of me, and I start to wonder why I have to manage this condition. "What did I ever do to deserve it?", sometimes I need to look myself in the mirror and say, "You did nothing. It's just part of your life. You will be able to manage it...stay healthy!"

One of the biggest steps forward I took when learning how to manage my condition was connecting with other women. I sought out PCOS groups on different social media channels, such as Facebook and Instagram. I also went to various websites where you can sign up to become part of the Forum. There are several places, such as pcoschallenge.org, that allow you to meet thousands of women who understand your experience. I found women who told me that what I was feeling was normal, and not to be ashamed. They continued to support me through the process with their advice, and by just lending me a hand or a place to vent or cry.

I was conscious that I had to achieve another goal: make some lifestyle changes.

I don't like changes to much, especially when I'm involved therefore, this was a step I took slowly. I gradually made changes, starting with my diet, because stay healthy it's one of the most important factors with this syndrome. I then focused on setting a better sleeping schedule, made sure I went to my medical check-ups, and practiced good self-care. I learned which self-care strategies were the best for my mental health so, I could overcome depression and anxiety, which are two psychological disorders that tend to attach women with PCOS.

In this book I'll explain what PCOS is and I'll give you tips to help you manage your symptoms and help you understand the links and battles between weight, inflammation, and insulin resistance. Then, we will start focusing on building a healthier diet by giving you dozens of amazing recipes that are suitable for you.

Let's focus on coming together through this journey, so we all know that no one is alone.

Chapter 1: What You Need to Know About PCOS

PCOS is a health condition in women that usually manifests during their childbearing years. It results in a hormonal imbalance, which can cause a lot of health issues, especially problems with fertility. It happens when your ovaries produce an abnormal amount of androgens, which are usually more present in men than women. Until recently, it's been a disease that hasn't received much awareness, although many researchers believe they can trace the first known case back to the 1700s (Harrar, 2017). However, this doesn't mean that physicians continued to monitor or research the disease. According to scientific standards, its research is still in the beginning stages.

Many women feel they are alone once diagnosed, but PCOS affects about 1 out of 10 women, which is 5 to 10% of the population (Reproductive Facts, 2014). According to the Centers for Disease Control and Prevention (CDC), PCOS affects about 5 million women. This number has increased dramatically over the last few decades, as more people have become aware of the disease. You usually receive a diagnosis in your 20s, but it's possible to be diagnosed in your teenage years or 30s as well.

When you're diagnosed, one of the first statements you'll hear from your doctor is that you're insulin-resistant. While your body makes insulin, it can't effectively use it, which makes you more susceptible to Type 2 Diabetes. Therefore, you want to put yourself on a specific diet. You also want to increase your amount of exercise, and take care of yourself by ensuring you communicate with your doctor and go to your annual checkups.

Common Signs and Symptoms

One of the biggest problems with diagnosing is that every woman will have different symptoms. Some will quickly go to the doctor since they're struggling with their health, while other women will barely notice any symptoms. In fact, you might have found out you have PCOS during a regular checkup. Other symptoms that might bring you to the doctor include:

Irregular periods. This is one of the most common signs of PCOS, but it's also common in females who are overweight, have thyroid issues, don't eat a healthy diet, don't exercise regularly, or have other health issues.

Acne. It's normal to have acne in your teens and early-20s because of your hormones and excess oil on your skin. Usually by your mid-20s, you'll start to notice your acne decreasing or disappearing nearly completely, at least for most of the month. It's also common for many women to deal with it during their menstrual cycle. Another sign is you have acne on your back, legs, chest, and neck. If you notice that you struggle with acne constantly and have other symptoms on this list, you should consult your doctor.

Increased growth of facial and body hair. The medical term for this is "hirsutism," and it is a symptom that you want to be weary of. Let's say it—the more you age, the more you'll notice unwanted facial and body hair. You start getting it in the regular places during puberty, and then it seems that your adult years can also bring more facial hair than you'd like to admit. This growth is normal for women, and you shouldn't worry about the few added hairs on your chin. The time to become concerned that you might have PCOS is when you have hair where men generally have hair on their body and face. If you start noticing a little more than a few hairs on your chin, or sideburns are showing more than normal, and you're experiencing other symptoms, talk to your physician during your next checkup.

Hair loss. This is another area that you probably don't like to talk and think about. For most women, hair is one of the best features. You take pride in your hair, so when it starts thinning out, you start to become more self-conscios. It's normal to associate this with aging, but you also need to be aware it's a common symptom of PCOS.

Sleeping problems. One reason many women go undiagnosed with the condition is because many of its symptoms can be blamed on other parts of life, such as trouble sleeping or feeling tired all of the time. You're busy with work, school, taking care of your family, or running a household. Plus, it seems that you always need to focus on other tasks apart from your job and your home, such as helping family, friends, shopping, and running errands. It's no secret that nearly every mom and wife usually feels a bit tired, but you shouldn't always contribute it to your busy lifestyle. In reality, you shouldn't have to spend your days feeling like a zombie or overtired. If you feel like you're stuck in a sleepless cycle, look at any other signs of PCOS and talk to your doctor.

Trouble getting pregnant. This is one of the reasons why most women with PCOS make their way to the doctor and find out about their condition. They've been trying to get pregnant for a while, sometimes years, and they're finally wanting to know if something is causing their infertility. For many people, this is the worst symptom because they long for a baby and feel that they don't have a chance—this is a myth. The truth is, you *can* get pregnant with PCOS, it might just be a bit harder. It's important not to lose faith when it comes to this sign, and talk to your doctor about how you can overcome it.

Weight gain. Whether you've always been a bit on the heavier side or notice you're starting to gain weight rapidly, you should contact your doctor if you have weight gain and other symptoms. If you've been trying to lose weight and following a diet, but still find yourself at the same or gaining weight, you could have PCOS. Fortunately, once you get on the right diet, you will start to notice the pounds shedding right off.

It's important to contact your physician if you feel you might of PCOS, because it can lead to a variety of other health issues:

- Gestational diabetes, when and if you do become pregnant, which puts you into a high risk pregnancy.
- High blood pressure, which can cause problems with other organs, such as the brain, kidneys, and heart.
- You're at a higher risk for heart disease and stroke, especially later in life.
- You could have trouble with sleep apnea, which causes you to randomly stop breathing during the night and leads to other health problems, such as diabetes and heart disease.

Mental health is also important to focus on with the syndrome. You're more likely to feel depressed or anxious. Researchers don't fully understand why, and they continue to monitor and study the link, but they do know there is a correlation.

What Causes PCOS?

You know the symptoms that you need to watch out for, but now you wonder, is there something that you can do to limit your chances of developing the disease? Why does it affect some women, but not others? If you're overweight, you have a higher chance of developing PCOS, especially if your body struggles to produce insulin.

Another cause is genes. You might have a mother, grandmother, or aunt who was diagnosed. According to studies, this increases your chances because it's known to run in families. However, scientists are still working on trying to understand what gene or genes are linked to the disease.

Inflammation is a big problem when it comes to the syndrome so many researchers feel this is one of the leading causes. There are several factors that can lead to your body becoming more inflamed in certain areas, such as your internal organs. It's normal for your body to have some swelling, but if you don't take care of yourself, it can lead to diseases. The best step to take is to eat foods that are known to decrease inflammation, such as whole grains, blueberries, green tea, turmeric, broccoli, avocado, and tomato. The key is to decrease it enough so that your white blood cells have more energy to fight off infections that come into your body.

It's important to note that doctors don't fully understand all of the causes, because the research is still in its infancy. When it comes to the greater causes, researchers believe they're on the right track but any study they conduct can add or change information. You want to make sure that you keep up-to-date on the advances of PCOS so you get the best information as soon as it's reported.

Advice for Newly Diagnosed

You've been diagnosed, and now you're wondering what to do. There are so many emotions and questions. You wonder if you'll be able to have children. You're grateful that you have an answer explaining your symptoms, but worry about what your future holds. You want to get as much information as possible about your condition, but not sure where to turn.

The first step to take is to take a deep breath. It's never easy receiving a diagnosis, especially one that can turn your life upside down. But your condition is manageable, you will learn how to live with it to your full potential.

Second, you want to educate yourself on the topic. You can do this by talking to your doctor and other people who have the syndrome, as well as by reading books and articles. The key is to focus on the truth. Most of the information you'll read developed over the last several decades, so there will be a lot of myths that many people mistake as facts. You want to find reputable sources. However, don't push yourself to learn everything in one night. Take your time so you don't become overwhelmed.

Third, realize that your story will have differences. PCOS isn't a one size fits all condition. For example, you might find that you need to focus on walking over running when it comes to exercise.

Fourth, social media is a great way to meet other people with the disease, but you don't want to depend on Facebook or

Twitter for your information. Not everything you read on social media is true, and a lot of the information can become mixed with someone's opinion or personal belief. You also want to be aware of any websites that use scare tactics, such as telling you what foods you have to avoid if diagnosed.

Fifth, assemble a team of professionals, such as an OB/GYN and endocrinologist, to help you learn about the research. You want to ensure that they're willing to be on your team and will keep lines of communication open with you and each other. You also want to keep up on your doctor visits and let other physicians know that you have PCOS when they might not know.

Sixth, pay more attention to your health and labs. You want to make sure that you're eating the right foods to limit your chances of having high blood pressure and diabetes. You also want to keep track of your numbers to help you stay healthy.

Seven, do your best to manage your stress. When you feel overwhelmed, you can find yourself struggling when it comes to your diet, sleep, and staying healthy. All of this is important to manage with the disease. Find ways that will help you destress, such as walking in nature, meditating, and exercise.

Eight, find a support team, such as friends, family, and coworkers. It's always a good idea to ask around your city to see if there is a support group that meets or if your area has any events focused on the topic.

Finally, find an exercise routine that works for you and your health. You might need to increase your amount of exercising. Talk to your team of professionals to help you learn the best process for you.

Chapter 2: Some Tips to Overcome the Common PCOS Symptoms

Learning to manage PCOS focuses on several areas of your life. You might feel that you need to find a new normal, or change your lifestyle completely. This can be frustrating and frightening at the same time, especially if you're not comfortable with changes. Fortunately, there are a variety of tips you can incorporate into your life to overcome its symptoms.

Tips for Managing Your Emotional and Mental Health

Many people focus more on their physical health than emotional and mental health, but all aspects of your health are important – even the seemingly invisible aspects. You need to remember to keep your overall health in check, which means paying close attention to your stress, self-esteem, depression, and environment.

One of the toughest emotional times occurs when you hear your doctor say, "You have tested PCOS positive." You might have so many emotions soar through your body that you can't even separate them. You might be worried because of what little you know about the disease, or you might have anxiety because of the infertility myth. For a few moments, you'll struggle to keep up with what your doctor is saying, but soon you'll snap back into reality. You need to know that this initial reaction is absolutely normal and understandable. Don't tell yourself that you're being overdramatic. Let yourself go through the emotions you're feeling. You need to accept them, so you can work through them and strengthen your mental health.

Once you get through the initial reactions, you can start to focus on learning about PCOS. When you research, take your time so you comprehend everything you're reading. Try to relate the symptoms to your life, and then find ways to manage them. While you're learning, take a breath and analyze your emotional health.

There is little scientific research on how women diagnosed with the syndrome react emotionally and mentally, but one study shows they're more likely to receive a diagnosis of anxiety, depression, or bipolar disorder (Nature's Best, n.d.). Some people say they feel sad because they know that something is wrong with their body and they can't fix it. Others state that they become depressed because they struggle managing their symptoms and feel they can't be the person they want to be. Another reason that mental illness is more common for women with PCOS is because of the irregular menstrual cycle. It's stressful for them, because they don't know when they're most likely to become pregnant or because their emotions become surprisingly unbalanced.

If you're feeling down for a few days, you should contact your doctor. They can refer you to a therapist who will help you learn more about your mental health, and how to manage your psychological response to your diagnosis. Some of the tips they will discuss are below.

- Realize that the emotions you're feeling are normal. There is nothing wrong with the worry, or sadness. Your feelings don't define who you are, they're simply letting you know how you feel about your new diagnosis.
- Don't ignore the negative emotions. You will feel anger, frustration, and so much more. It's easy you want to push these aside because you believe you're always supposed to be strong and positive. No matter how you're feeling, you need to accept it so you can learn how to manage it. The more you ignore your emotions, the worse your mental state will become. Negativity builds up inside of you, and you need to release it so you can bring in more positivity.
- Take time to be alone. Don't feel that you need to always be around your loved ones, especially when you're mentally struggling. When you take time to be by yourself, you get to sort through your emotions and learn more about yourself. This can guide you to understand how to manage your symptoms.

- Open up about your thoughts and emotions. If you don't want to talk to family, find support groups for PCOS online or in your community. You can also contact a therapist, as they're trained to help you through challenging moments in your life.
- Practice mindfulness. You might start to focus on meditation, or simply look at ways you can become more mindful. For example, spending time with nature to learn about its sounds and smells, or paying attention when you're eating, driving to work, and completing common household tasks. Notice what your hands are doing, what your thoughts are saying, and how you react to certain stimuli.
- Meditation can also help you destress, which is important for your diagnosis. If you feel that you're taking on too much, decrease your workload. You want to also learn how to say "no," and realize that you don't need a reason to tell someone that you can't take on a new project or help them in that moment.
- Slow down and take a break when you start to feel anxious. Take a few deep and slow breaths, as this will decrease your heart rate and make you feel more relaxed.
- Find a hobby that you enjoy, such as painting, writing, putting puzzles together, or spending time with animals. You might find that volunteering at a local organization helps you feel happier and less stressed.

Tips for Managing Your Physical Health

When it comes to your physical health, one of the first tips you will receive from your doctor and anyone who lives with PCOS is to follow the diet strictly. You'll find yourself struggling, especially at first, with cravings. You need to have self-control so you can overcome these moments. One strategy is to use delayed gratification, which is when you resist temptation for as long as possible, or until it goes away. It's important to note that you might give into your cravings the first few times. When this happens, be gentle with yourself and continue to try the strategy. Over time, you'll notice that you delay the craving longer. Soon, you'll beat your cravings and stick to your diet more easily.

Another tip for sticking to your diet is ensuring you still get the necessary food groups in your everyday meals. Follow the advice of your doctors, and create a meal plan. Take time out of your week to go through meals you want to make the following week, and ensure that they're all balanced so you get all your vitamins and nutrients. You can also take time to prepare your meals, which will help you keep to your meal plan.

By following a specific diet, you'll decrease inflammation, help your hormones maintain balance, and keep yourself as healthy as possible. It's important to understand that when you have high inflammation in your body, you can easily become sick . You might find yourself struggling with the common cold and flu frequently. It will feel like every time you're around someone who is ill, you become ill as well. You'll also have a higher chance of diabetes and heart disease.

You'll hear a lot about insulin-resistance. One of the best ways to manage this is through your diet. You want to focus on obtaining a low glycemic index (GI) diet. The GI focuses on measuring how fast foods raise blood levels. Therefore, you'll eat foods that raise your levels slowly, so your insulin doesn't spike to an unhealthy level. Some of the best foods are vegetables, whole fruits, lean protein, whole wheat, and healthy fats. You will also want to eat more fiber, as this will slow down the digestive process and combat insulin resistance. You'll want to avoid foods that are high in sugar and/or processed. You can get a great start on your diet with the 100+ recipes in Chapter 8.

Losing weight can help you manage several of your physical PCOS symptoms. Not only will it help your hormones reach their natural levels, but it will also improve the way your body handles insulin, and lower your blood sugar glucose levels. Furthermore, a correct weight can help regulate your menstrual cycle and aid in the chances of you becoming pregnant.

Another way to help alleviate symptoms is by eating smaller meals throughout the day. You're used to eat about three larger meals and then snacking in-between, but it's better for your weight, hormone, and insulin levels to eat four to five smaller meals during the day. You can do this by cutting your regular-size portions in half.

Increase your exercises, but in a way that won't make you feel overwhelmed or exhausted quickly. When your body is struggling with PCOS, you can begin to feel tired easily, especially when your insulin and hormone levels aren't well balanced. You want to gradually add exercises into your routine. You also want to focus on a regimen that's easy on your body. For example, if you find that jogging or running is too difficult for you, start with walking, and then slowly bring yourself to jogging. You might realize that lifting weights tires you out quickly, so in that case you might want to include more cardio and yoga.

You don't need to exercise every day. In fact, you want to look at a weekly time frame instead of hours in a day or number of days. Most experts believe you should exercise at least 150 minutes every week. You can divide this into so many minutes every day, or 50 minutes three days a week. Another key is to realize that your body needs more nourishment during your highly active days. You want to focus more on energy-boosting foods and drinks, but keep the sugars low. For example, if you only allow yourself to eat so much protein during the week, eat more on your exercise days.

Chapter 3: The Battle Between PCOS and the Weight Scale

PCOS is like any other disorder; when you receive a diagnosis, it changes parts of your life. Your lifestyle and how you react to certain stimuli can change either drastically or over time. For example, you know that you need to follow a special diet; this change begins right away, but your increase in fitness might occur over time.

One of the biggest battles you'll face will be against the weight scale. Many women feel anxious before they get on the scale because they feel as though they need to watch their weight closely. This causes them to feel that when their weight increases normally, within a couple of pounds, they're doing something wrong with their diet. It's important to remember that weight fluctuates on a daily basis. For instance, if you skipped breakfast and then jumped on the scale before dinner you might see that you weigh a pound less than the previous morning, when you did have breakfast. It also depends on the clothing you wear, if you changed your shoes, and several other factors.

The most important piece of information for you is knowing how to keep the correct weight, which focuses on the body mass index (BMI) chart. It's a useful tool that helps you understand whether you are underweight, overweight, or at a healthy weight. Its main focus is your height, and while most experts follow it, there are shortcomings. For example, it doesn't take your gender, frame size, age, or muscle tone into count. You've probably seen the numbers before, and know exactly what the chart looks like. Your doctor might have had a conversation explaining where you are now and where you should be.

Other than your doctor's office, you can find a BMI chart online and even calculate at what point you should be at. Several websites, such as the World Cancer Research Fund and the Center for Disease Control and Prevention, have calculators where you simply add in your height and weight to see where you are on the chart.

It's important to not become discouraged if you find that you're not at a healthy weight. While you need to get your weight under control, there are several steps you can take to ensure you're as healthy as possible after diagnosis.

Increment Physical Activity

Even if you don't include much physical activity in your day, you can gradually change this to improve your health and PCOS symptoms. The key is to increase your activity rate slowly, and develop an exercise routine that works for you. For instance, if you have a heart disorder, you want to focus more on cardio exercises. If you have a lifestyle where setting aside time is a problem, you might find it beneficial to focus on exercises for 20 minutes in the morning and then 10 in the evening.

Another option is to get up and move more around your house or/and office. For example, set an alarm to remind you to get up every 45 minutes and walk around for five minutes, stretch, or take time to complete desk exercises.

If you have a fitbit, increase the number of steps you want to reach on a weekly basis. You might start with 5,000 every day, and then the next week go up to 6,000. You can even add a few hundred steps every time you reach your goal for four consecutive days.

You can also increase your activity by getting up to dance. You don't need to be a good dancer, you just need to have fun and move. If you feel like shutting the shades and closing the door to your office, do that. You can also talk to a coworker about joining you for a couple of quick dance sessions throughout the day, or if you're at home, have a little fun with your children or pets. You might even talk to your partner about learning different dances through YouTube videos.

If you're planning a date with your significant other, choose to be active. Instead of going out to eat and then to the movies (or deciding to stay in and watch Netflix) go for a walk, bike ride, take up salsa dancing, square dancing, bowling, or do anything that doesn't involve sitting in a chair for most of the evening. You could also decide to walk to your dinner date instead of driving.

Are you planning a meeting at work? If so, you can incorporate walk meetings. They don't always work well with large groups, but if you're meeting with your supervisor or business partner about an idea, you can easily walk around the block while you brainstorm. If you need to write something down, take out your phone and record it or send yourself an email.

If you have a desk job, you can find a way to stand at your desk instead of sit. You can go on Amazon and purchase a stand that allows you to move your screen up or down, get a laptop-standing desk, or get creative and make one yourself. You can also talk to your supervisor to see what options your company is willing to offer you.

Follow a Natural and Balanced PCOS Diet

One of the most important steps in managing your health is following a specific diet. Don't let the word "diet" frighten you, because it's easier to incorporate it into your life more than you think. Plus, your diet can be filled with a variety of yummy foods to help keep your body and mind strong.

There is a myth that states you can follow the Ketogenic diet. It's important to note that there are many ideas that are similar, such as eating healthy fats (oils, avocado, eggs, fish, and nuts). However, there is no scientific proof that Keto will help you ease your symptoms, and this is one of the main reasons why you'd want to change your eating lifestyle.

You don't want to follow a meal plan that will limit your caloric intake. Taking this approach would be like grabbing the wrong tool for the job. You need to focus on eating foods that will help your insulin resistance. You also don't want to aim for a plant-based diet, because eggs and fish have nine essential amino acids that you need to help fight your symptoms. If you're vegan or can't eat dairy products, you must speak with your doctor so they can help you get the nutrients that you need. If you have a high amount of healthy fats in your diet, you can decrease the number of carbs you eat, but don't limit yourself to as low as 15%. It's best to stay around the 20 to 30% range.

Another tip when it comes to maintaining a healthy diet is this: your biggest meal should be breakfast. You can have a larger lunch or dinner, but not both. For instance, you eat a bigger breakfast and evening meal, and have three other smaller dishes throughout the day. The reason you want to focus on your first meal is because it can help you regulate and balance your hormones.

It won't be easy, but you want to do your best to eliminate sugar as well. The fact is, sugar can make certain symptoms worse. It's known to make facial hair grow in places you don't want them to grow, increase your amount of acne, and make your body more likely to store fat instead of burn it.

The healthiest diet for you would include focusing on eggs, meat, and fish. Eating these foods will help you stay full longer, because they're high in protein. You want to curb your hunger pains by eating foods that will silence them, not slightly decrease them like carbohydrates and sugar do. High protein foods will help you cut any snacking between your meals.

Another tip to help you keep your PCOS diet balanced is to eliminate vegetable oil. Yes, it's a common ingredient that many use because it's a good high-fat ingredient. In reality, there are a lot of trans fats in vegetable oil, which are bad for you. It's also known to increase inflammation in your body, which will make your symptoms worse.

You want to add a lot of non-starchy vegetables into your diet, such as carrots, broccoli, asparagus, radishes, cauliflower, cucumber, onions, and peppers. You can eat as many as you want throughout the day, and it's okay to have some for every meal. For example, you might have broccoli with eggs in the morning, carrot sticks for a snack, a salad for lunch, and then have mixed vegetables in the evening as a side.

Finally, to help you maintain a diet (especially in the beginning, when it can be challenging), you should contact a nutritionist. They can become a part of your professional care team and help you focus on meals that are right for you. They will also help you set up meal plans, and even give you advice on meal preparations so you're not tempted to buy quick, unhealthy, and processed foods.

Chapter 4: Having PCOS Doesn't Mean You're Infertile

One of the biggest myths about PCOS is that you can't become pregnant. This is one reason many women emotionally struggle when they're first diagnosed. They've been trying to get pregnant for several months, and now are told they have a disease that makes them infertile. But this isn't true. You need to realize that having PCOS doesn't mean you're infertile. In fact, there are thousands of women with the syndrome who never have a problem becoming pregnant.

Ovulation in Women

By now, you know that you have about a three day window when it comes to getting pregnant. You know that you need to know when you're ovulating, so you have a higher chance of conceiving. The problem for you is that your menstrual cycle isn't regular, so how can you be sure when you're ovulating?

Usually, a menstrual cycle occurs when certain hormones secrete in the brain, telling an egg follicle located in the ovary to start developing. PCOS affects this process because of the amount of androgens your body produces. It's possible for your egg to start growing, but then not mature, which means it won't get released. In response, your body won't continue the menstrual cycle at that time. Your brain can communicate with the egg again a couple of weeks later, but you might follow the same process. It might be a couple of months before you go through a complete cycle. You also have the possibility of a longer than average period. They can also be heavier than average, and cause more pain.

An irregular cycle is frustrating when you're trying to get pregnant, or simply want to feel prepared for that time. Fortunately, there are signs that you're heading into ovulation, including:

Basal body temperature (BBT). Start charting your temperature when you wake up every morning. When you're close to ovulating, you will have a higher temperature. The key is to record your numbers at the same time every morning. Set a digital thermometer and a way to record the numbers right by your bed. There are a number of apps that you can download to your cell phone or tablet, such as Glow Cycle & Fertility Tracker, Flo Period & Ovulation Tracker, and Natural Cycles. You will start to notice your temperature rising slowly over a few days. When you notice the trend, you'll be ovulating soon. Once you drop back down to normal, you're no longer ovulating.

Checking your cervix. During your menstrual cycle, your cervix changes position. When you're close to ovulating, it's in a higher position and harder to find. Another change to consider is the mucus. You'll be dry at the start of your cycle but it will change to a raw egg type texture when your body is getting ready to ovulate.

Ovulation prediction kits. There are many natural ways to know when you're heading toward ovulation, but you can also purchase a kit to help you. Many people pick up a couple of kits when they start tracking so they have a peace of mind. The kits look for elevated levels of luteinizing hormone (LH). The higher the level, the closer you are to ovulation. Before you go out and buy, you need to realize that your LH levels are naturally higher because of PCOS, so they might not be as effective.

Being Pregnant with PCOS

Once you become pregnant, you'll learn there are different risks involved because of your disease. It's important to listen to the advice of your medical team, so you can ensure that your baby is born healthy and you don't have to worry about complications. At the same time, they'll inform you about any preparations that you need to consider. Don't let your mind make you worry too much, because your doctors have you and your baby's best interest at heart.

At this point, if you haven't found a support group yet, I highly encourage you to. Your mind can cause a lot of anxiety when it comes to your pregnancy, plus you'll have changes in your hormonal balance which can cause more challenges mentally, emotionally, and physically. Find women through Facebook groups that were pregnant with PCOS. They will help you by sharing their stories and giving you advice.

You'll be considered a high risk pregnancy because you have higher chances of premature birth, high blood pressure, gestational diabetes, and miscarriage. Another condition that you'll learn about is preeclampsia. There are four main symptoms: high blood pressure, protein in urine, excessive weight gain, and swelling of hands and feet. It can cause damage to your organs, especially liver and kidneys. If you're diagnosed with it at any point during your pregnancy, you'll be watched carefully. Your doctor appointments will increase, you might be placed on bed rest, and you might end up staying in the hospital until you deliver. It's more likely you'll have a cesarean delivery due to complications or the size of your baby.

Other than a higher chance of complications, your pregnancy will be similar to women without PCOS. By following your doctor's orders, ensuring you eat a healthy diet and get all the nutrients that you and your baby need, and not letting stress or other negative emotions affect you, you'll decrease your chances of complications.

Chapter 5: The Relationship Between PCOS and Chronic Inflammation

Inflammation is a natural part of your body's immune system. You'll have a little bit of it in your body at times and not even know it. Usually it's a sign that you're about to get sick, or that your body is trying to fight off an infection. Unfortunately, inflammation can quickly increase or become chronic, and you might find yourself struggling with diseases and illnesses, such as a common cold, cancer, or PCOS. Your immune system might also be triggered to react to its own cells and tissues, including ones that are meant to keep you healthy, in response to inflammation.

When you have the syndrome, it's common to have low-grade chronic inflammation, which is one reason you are at an increased risk for type 2 diabetes and coronary heart disease. It's important to note that studies show heart disease as being more prevalent with your inflammation than type 2 diabetes (Kelly et al., 2001).

Symptoms of Chronic Inflammation

One of the best ways to help lower chronic inflammation is to understand its symptoms, so you can contact your doctor for help as soon as possible. When you get to this type of inflammation, your immune system can remain inflamed for months or years. This gives you different signs than other types. These signs include:

Fatigue. Most people don't think of fatigue as a symptom for chronic inflammation, but it's one of the common ones. The struggle is, you think that you're constantly tired because you have a busy lifestyle. You might have a full-time job, family, and maybe going to college. You're bringing your children to different extracurricular activities while trying to make everyone a healthy evening meal at the same time. Your days cause you to feel stress, which can escalate your tiredness. The trick is to go through how well you sleep at night and how busy you are. If you find that you're not getting seven to eight hours of good sleep every night, focus on changing this. If you still feel tired after sleeping well, notice any other symptoms on this list you have and consult your doctor.

Body pain. This is probably one of the most notable signs. You understand that pain is often caused from inflammation, so you need to take certain medications to help it decrease. For example, you take Ibuprofen for a headache. But the types of discomforts you need to focus on for PCOS is joint and muscle aches. You might also feel random abdominal pain that you don't understand. It might be like menstrual cramps, but not as strong.

Skin rashes. You can get rashes around the site of your pain, or anywhere else. They're characterized by flaky, red, itchy skin. It's common to have them on your hands, legs, arms, and stomach. Rashes, such as eczema and psoriasis, are connected to the immune system; this makes them common for those with PCOS.

Gastrointestinal complications. If you suffer from stomach problems, diarrhea, or constipation, you might have inflammation in your digestive tract. It can show itself as Inflammatory Bowel Disease (IBD) and carry its own symptoms. You should note that you can have IBD and not have PCOS, but only a doctor can determine this.

Depression and anxiety. When you're tired all of the time and not feeling well, your mental and emotional health becomes affected. You don't understand why you're feeling unwell, but you know something is wrong, and this leads you to worry about your health or become depressed.

Excessive mucus production. Do you feel like you need to clear your throat often? Are you constantly blowing your nose? Do you feel that you have more mucus in your body than normal? It's a common symptom for PCOS, because it's also a sign of inflammation.

Tips to Control Inflammation

There are many questions about which diet is best for PCOS. Some people say that it's best to stick to foods that will help decrease chronic inflammation and other symptoms. Therefore, professionals are looking into creating a diet that is specific for your condition. However, many studies show that the Mediterranean diet can also be helpful in decreasing inflammation, leading many people to believe it's one of the best for those with PCOS at this time.

The Mediterranean diet focuses on foods that you will find along the coasts of the Mediterranean. It's based on fruits, poultry, vegetables, fish, nuts, beans, whole grains, herbs, and healthy oils (olive, avocado, coconut, and sesame). You will also eat moderate amounts of eggs and other dairy products, but they're not as common as other diets. You can eat small amounts of red meat. What this means is that you want to limit it to about once a week. You want to stay away from unhealthy fats, processed foods, greasy foods, and sweets.

Another tip is to limit or stop drinking alcohol. While many people say a glass of wine now and then is fine, you don't want to find yourself having a glass every day. Instead of wine, turn yourself toward water, sprinkling water, or another healthy drink. If you're used to having wine with dinner, put your beverage in a wine glass as this will help your mind make the transfer to a non-alcoholic drink.

You want to take time to exercise, but you don't want to overdo it. It's possible to increase your inflammation if you push your body too much. Start with what you can do and then slowly increase your routine. For example, if you only go for a 20 minute walk every day, start by adding five minutes. A few days later you can look at going on a treadmill for a few minutes and then gradually increase this time. Look for other avenues that won't cause you to push yourself too much, such as Yoga or a few cardio exercises.

Keep your stress in check. It's easier said than done, but your health depends on limiting your stress as much as possible. If you need to reach out for help, don't be ashamed to consult a therapist. They can help you understand where most of your stress is coming from and what you can do to change it. They can also show you strategies, such as deep breathing exercises, to help you manage your stress level.

Finally, make sure you get yourself on a good sleep schedule. This can not only help you manage your stress, but it can make you feel better overall. You'll find yourself thinking more clearly and being able to focus better. You'll want to eat healthier meals. When you feel better mentally, you'll take care of yourself better physically.

Chapter 6: The Link Between PCOS and Insulin Resistance

You know that insulin resistance is one of the biggest indicators of people with PCOS. It happens when your liver, fat, and muscles don't communicate well with your insulin. This makes it harder for them to use your glucose from your blood to create energy. While the scientific studies are still in its infancy, many show that there is a strong link between the two, and that it's one reason why you have the symptoms that you do.

Naturally, the risk for insulin resistance is higher for women who are over the age of 40, overweight, have high cholesterol, and high blood pressure. If you don't pay attention to your diet, you get poor sleep, and you don't exercise regularly, you also increase your chances of developing resistance.

Symptoms of Insulin Resistance

One symptom is craving sweets. This is more than just having a "sweet tooth," which you might have had all of your life. You will feel the cravings come on as you age, and they can get to the point where you can't say "no." You feel that you need to have a slice of pie, brownie, or even a few pieces of chocolate because you can't get your mind away from the thought. You feel like you're drooling at the sight of the sweets.

Along with sugar type foods and drinks, you'll also crave salt. You might find that your favorite new snack is trail mix, because you get the sweet and salty at the same time. You might go from eating a few M&Ms to having a handful of chips.

One of the most notable signs is that certain parts of your skin starts to darken. You'll notice this specifically around your armpits, groin, or behind the neck. It doesn't come on quickly, but you probably won't realize that your skin is slowly getting darker. Instead, you'll be taking a shower or look in the mirror and notice a difference in color.

Other symptoms are tingling of hands and feet, feeling hungry even after you've eaten a full meal, and extreme thirst. You will also feel more tired than normal, and make frequent trips to the bathroom as you feel that you need to urinate. This ties in with drinking more than your usual amount of fluids, but it also has to do with the way your body is handling your insulin. You will also find yourself becoming more ill than usual with the common cold, or other diseases going around. Even if you receive the flu shot, you can still find yourself sick with influenza even months after the fact.

Understanding the Glycemic Index

The glycemic index (GI) is a tool that you can use when considering which foods to eat; it will help you manage your blood sugar. It consists of several factors, such as the cooking method you use for food, the amount of time the food is processed, its nutrient composition, and its ripeness. For instance, a banana will have a higher GI when it's ripe. You can also lower the number when you boil foods. There are many benefits to following this tool, as it can also help you lose weight and reduce your cholesterol.

There are three ratings to use when referring to this index. When your GI is low, you're at a 55 or less. Medium is 56 to 69, and high is 70 and above. You want to focus on eating foods in the lower category. While you can go into the other two areas, it's important to limit the amount of food you consume.

How do you know when you're eating foods that are in the high category? Because they're high in refined carbohydrates and sugars. They also have a higher unhealthy fat content. So, you want to focus on foods that follow the Mediterranean or an insulin resistance diet.

To give you an idea of certain foods and their GI content, here are some of the most common that you'll eat on a regular basis:

Fruit:

- Strawberry: 41

- Banana: 51
- Watermelon: 76
- Pineapple: 59
- Mango: 51
- Apple: 36
- Orange: 43
- Blueberry: 53

Grains:

- Quinoa: 53
- Popcorn: 65
- White rice: 73
- Barley: 28
- Rolled oats: 55
- White bread: 75
- Whole wheat bread: 74
- Brown rice: 68

Vegetables (boiled):

- Potato: 78
- Sweet potato: 63
- Pumpkin: 74
- Carrots: 39
- Broccoli: 15
- Chickpeas: 33
- Asparagus: 15
- Cucumber: 15
- Tomato: 15
- Lettuce: 15

- Sweet corn: 54

Dairy:

- Skim milk: 37
- Ice cream: 51
- Rice milk: 86
- Soymilk: 34
- Whole milk: 39
- Low-fat yogurt: 14
- Fruit yogurt: 36
- Chocolate milk: 35
- Plain yogurt: 14

Beans:

- Kidney beans: 41
- Pinto beans: 55
- Dried beans: 40
- Split peas: 45
- Black-eyed beans: 59

Sweeteners:

- Coconut sugar: 54
- Table sugar: 65
- Honey: 61
- Fructose: 15
- Maple syrup: 54

Chapter 7: Food as a Medicine: A National Balanced and Insulin Resistant Diet

The insulin resistance diet used to focus on people who were diabetic, but research shows that it's a healthy way for people with PCOS to eat. The key is to focus on making sure you're eating the right foods and maintaining the right balance. This is actually easier than it sounds, because you don't focus on needing to make special foods. Instead, you focus on avoiding sugar, red meats, processed starches, unhealthy fats, and vegetables that are high in GI content. You want to aim for foods that are whole grains, lean poultry, fruits, vegetables low in GI content or boiled, and fish.

Foods to Consume

You should have 5 to 15 servings of fruits a day. You can consume any of them, such as mangoes, plantains, pears, berries, all melons, nectarines, dates, tangerines, apples, oranges, etc.

You also want to eat at least ½ of head to 1 head every day of your greens. These include kale, arugula, cabbage varieties, lettuce, and chard.

It's important to include one to three servings of whole grains in your daily diet, such as brown, wild, and black rice. You can also eat oats, barley, corn, rye, buckwheat, quinoa, and amaranth.

Many people feel it's best to eat more non-starchy vegetables than starchy ones. But, when it comes to this food group, you need to have two to five servings per day. You can mix several into your meals and snack by including cucumbers, onions, carrots, celery, mushrooms, bell peppers, cauliflower, and artichokes. Starchy vegetables that are safe to consume include, but are not limited to, squash varieties, potato varieties, yams, turnips, and parsnips.

There are some vegetables that are referred to as nightshades. These are ones that contain alkaloids, which can trigger inflammation in some people. While you can eat them, you want to notice how you feel afterwards. If you notice that you have more signs of inflammation over the next couple of days, limit them. Otherwise, you should eat about five servings a day. These include hot peppers, sweet peppers, white potatoes, tomatoes, pepinos, paprika, and eggplant.

You don't want to forget about your legumes, which consist of one to three servings per day. For example, soy yogurt, all varieties of beans, soy products, all varieties of peas, and all varieties of lentils.

You shouldn't have a problem including at least two servings of spices and herbs into your diet, because you'll use them to help improve the taste of your food. Some of the best to keep in your cupboard are cinnamon, cumin, cardamom, garlic, turmeric, ginger, fennel, thyme, balis, oregano, and rosemary. While you can also use salt, most people like to stick to sea salt.

Foods to Limit

When it comes to limiting foods, you want to have zero to one serving a day. Usually, it's best to keep it to a few throughout the week, but it's also up to how your body reacts to the ingredients. If you ever notice that your inflammation increases, you should stop consuming these foods at all. Everyone reacts differently to many foods, so you want to ensure that you're always paying attention to signs.

Conventional pastas are ones you should keep to zero to two servings per week. They include spaghetti, penne, fettuccine, whole wheat pasta, semolina pasta, and lasagne.

Nuts are always a good idea to add to your meals, especially when you're looking for a unique taste or an added crunch. But you also want to limit them because they can cause higher rates of inflammation. These include cashews, pistachios, walnuts, macadamia nuts, almonds, brazil nuts, hazelnuts, pine nuts, pecans, and peanuts.

Along with nuts, you want to limit seeds in your daily diet. You should keep sunflower, sesame, chia, flax, and hemp seeds to between zero to one serving.

Granola and fatty plants, such as coconuts, olives, durian, and avocados, should also be limited.

Foods to Avoid

It's hard to completely avoid foods, especially when you love the ones in this category. But, the more you stay away from them, the better you will feel. In reality, you don't need to look at this as foods you can never have, especially as snacks or with your meals ever again. The key is to limit them to once a month or less. You also don't want to eat several of these foods in the same time frame. For example, if you know you'll have to accompany your child to a birthday party next week, stay away from these foods so you can have a small piece of cake at the party.

The biggest type of food to avoid is sweets and sweetened drinks, such as sodas and vitamin water. This also includes juices that aren't freshly squeezed. You should also avoid trans and saturated fats, also known as bad fats. Another area to stay away from is processed foods.

Tips for a Healthy Diet

Build your self-control. Let's get down to the foundation of a healthy diet: your self-discipline. It's that part of you that makes you get up so you're not late for work. You want to listen to this side of you when it comes to keeping your diet healthy. Most people struggle with self-control when it comes to food, especially when they love the taste. If you have a bit of a sweet tooth or love your fast food, you'll want to use strategies to help build your discipline so you're not eating these foods too often. For example, when you're craving a brownie, you might grab an apple instead. You can also develop a meal plan every week to keep you from thinking you need to go through McDonald's because it's faster than making food at home.

Don't skip meals. If you ever heard that missing a meal can help you lose weight because you're eating less food during the day, you heard wrong. The reality is that your metabolism needs to continue working to help you lose weight. Therefore, you need to keep it active through exercises or eating throughout the day. This is one reason why experts will tell you to eat smaller meals, but more of them, throughout the day.

Look at calories, but don't be obsessed. It's okay to focus on foods that are low-calorie, but some of them you shouldn't eat often. You want to focus on foods that will help you insulin resistance more than limit the amount of calories. You can make a plan to only eat the regular 2,000 calories a day or a little less, but don't fall into the trap of "it's low calories or nothing."

Fill up on vegetables and fruits. Of course, you want to eat a balanced diet, but most of the foods you will consume come from these two food groups, so fill up on them. Add more broccoli into your dinner so you eat less poultry. Pick up a piece of fruit or grab a handful of baby carrots if you want a snack.

Try the Mediterranean Diet. If you like the main food groups from this type of diet, try it. You might find that it suits you better than focusing on a specific insulin resistance diet, and you receive the same benefits. Pay attention to your body and you won't have a problem learning what foods you can eat often and what ones to limit.

Look for lean meats. Unless you're vegetarian or vegan, you will have meat in your diet. The best ones to have are the ones that are lean, such as chicken and turkey. If you choose to have red meat once a week, choose the types that have less fat and are more lean.

Chapter 8: Recipes

The following variety of recipes–ranging from Breakfast to Lunch and Dinner to Snacks and Sides and everything in between–are included so that you can get a jump-start on your new diet! Enjoy, and happy cooking!

Breakfast

Kale and Pepper Egg Bake

Prep time: 10 minutes

Cook time: 30 minutes

Serving size: 4

Nutritional information: Calories-224; Carbs-15 grams; Fat-13 grams; Protein-15 grams

Ingredients:

- 8 eggs
- 1 chopped sweet onion

- 1 chopped bell pepper
- ½ minced jalapeno pepper
- 4 cups chopped spinach
- 1 tablespoon olive oil
- 2 teaspoons minced garlic
- 1 tablespoon chopped fresh basil
- sea salt and ground black pepper for seasoning

Directions:

1. Preheat your oven to 375°F.
2. Place an oven-safe skillet on medium heat and pour in the olive oil.
3. Sauté onions and garlic until soft.
4. Combine peppers and sauté for 3 minutes.
5. Add spinach and sauté until wilted.
6. In a bowl, whisk the eggs, basil, salt, and pepper.
7. Pour egg mixture into the skillet. Stir thoroughly.
8. Set the skillet into the oven and time for 20 minutes.

Microwavable Egg Veggie Breakfast

Prep time: 2 to 3 minutes

Cook time: 1 to 2 minutes

Serving size: 1

Nutritional information: Calories-201; Carbs-12 grams; Fats-5 grams; Protein-6 grams

Ingredients:

- 2 tablespoons chopped mushrooms
- 2 eggs
- 2 tablespoons sliced baby spinach
- 1 tablespoon water
- A few sliced cherry tomatoes or grapes
- Serve with a ½ cup strawberries

Directions:

1. Spray a microwavable-safe dish with olive oil or cooking spray.
2. Whisk the egg, spinach, water, and mushrooms. Blend well.
3. Cover the bowl with a paper towel and place in the microwave for 30 seconds.
4. Carefully remove the bowl and stir.
5. Place back in the microwave for another 30 to 45 seconds, or until the egg is cooked thoroughly.
6. Top with the grapes or tomatoes.
7. Serve with strawberries on the side.

Navy Bean Egg Scramble

Prep time: 10 minutes

Cook time: 15 minutes

Serving size: 4

Nutritional information: Calories-333; Carbs-28 grams; Fat-13 grams; Protein-20 grams

Ingredients:

- 8 whisked eggs
- 2 cups navy beans (sodium-free is best), drained and rinsed
- ½ diced avocado
- 2 teaspoons olive oil
- ½ cup salsa
- 1 tablespoon cilantro, fresh and chopped

Directions:

1. Set a large skillet over medium heat and pour in the olive oil.
2. Once the oil is warm, add the beans and sauté for five minutes.
3. Combine the eggs. As they started to harden, pull them around the skillet with the spatula to scramble them.
4. Top with salsa, avocado, and cilantro.

Summer Eggs in a Pan

Prep time: 5 minutes

Cook time: 10 minutes

Serving size: 2

Nutritional information: Calories-255; Carbs-13 grams; Fat-6 grams; Protein-9 grams

Ingredients:

- 2 large zucchini
- 4 eggs
- 1 crushed garlic clove
- 1 tablespoon olive oil
- 1 pack (7 oz.) cherry tomatoes, halved
- Basil to serve

Directions:

1. Place a non-stick skillet over medium heat.
2. Pour in the olive oil and allow it to heat up.
3. Add the zucchini and fry for 5 minutes, stirring regularly.
4. Combine the garlic and tomatoes and cook for another 2 minutes.
5. Make two gaps in the mix and add 2 eggs into each gap.
6. Cover the pan and cook for another 3 minutes or until the eggs are done.
7. Scatter basil over the top and serve.

Egg Casserole with Sweet Potato

Prep time: 10 minutes

Cook time: 50 minutes

Serving size: 4

Nutritional information: Calories-183; Carbs-16 grams; Fat-9 grams; Protein-10 grams

Ingredients:

- 1 chopped onion
- 6 eggs
- 2 diced sweet potatoes
- 3 teaspoons olive oil
- 2 teaspoons minced garlic
- Sea salt and pepper for seasoning

Directions:

1. Turn your oven to 350°F.
2. Use 1 tablespoon olive oil to grease an 8 by 8-inch pan.
3. Pour the rest of the oil into a large skillet and place over medium heat.
4. Combine the potatoes, garlic, and onion. Sauté for 7 to 10 minutes.
5. Spread mixture into the pan.
6. Whisk the eggs and seasonings in a bowl and pour them on top of the mixture.

7. Set in the oven and bake for 40 minutes, or until the edges are crisp.

Citrus Pineapple Smoothie

Prep time: 5 minutes

Cook time: none

Serving size: 2

Nutritional information: Calories-273, Carbs-43 grams, Fat-5 grams, Protein-3 grams

Ingredients:

- 1 ½ cups frozen or fresh pineapple chunks
- 1 banana
- Juice from one lime
- 1 peeled and quartered orange
- 1 tablespoon ginger
- 2 teaspoons turmeric
- ¾ cup water
- 4 ice cubes
- ½ teaspoon nutmeg
- ½ cup coconut milk

Directions:

1. Combine all the ingredients into a blender and mix until smooth.
2. Add more water to get your desired consistency

Breakfast Smoothie

Prep time: 5 minutes

Cook time: none

Serving size: 1

Nutritional information: Calories-192; Carbs-39 grams; Fat-1 gram; Protein-8 grams

Ingredients:

- 1 can of peaches (with the juice)
- 2 bananas
- 1 ½ cup of raspberries, you can also use blueberries or blackberries
- 1 cup Greek yogurt
- ½ cup rolled oats
- 3 ice cubes

Directions:

1. Combine all the ingredients into a blender and mix until it has a smooth consistency.
2. If it's too thick, add a little water.

PB&J Smoothie

Prep time: 5 minutes

Cook time: none

Serving size: 1

Nutritional information: Calories-274; Carbs-16 grams; Fat-20 grams; Protein-12 grams

Ingredients:

- ½ cup sliced strawberries
- 1 cup unsweetened almond milk
- 1 teaspoon raw honey
- 2 tablespoon natural peanut butter
- 3 ice cubes

Directions:

1. Combine all the ingredients except the ice cubes and blend until the consistency is smooth.
2. Add the ice cubes and blend well.

3. Add some water for desired consistency.

Cherry Chocolate and Cinnamon Smoothie

Prep time: 3 to 4 minutes

Cook time: none

Serving size: 2

Nutritional information: Calories-235; Carbs-33 grams; Fats-4 grams; Protein-3 grams

Ingredients:

- 1 banana
- 2 tablespoons unsweetened cocoa powder
- ½ cup coconut milk
- 1 ½ cups frozen or fresh cherries
- ¾ cup water
- 2 teaspoons cinnamon
- 4 ice cubes

Directions:

1. Combine all of the ingredients into a blender and mix until smooth.

Green Tea Pear Smoothie

Prep time: 5 minutes

Cook time: none

Serving size: 2

Nutritional information: Calories-211, Carbs-20 grams, Fat-15 grams, Protein-3 grams

Ingredients:

- ½ cup unsweetened coconut milk
- ½ cup cold brewed green tea
- 1 cored pear
- 1 teaspoon raw honey
- ½ cup chopped swiss chard
- ½ teaspoons ground cinnamon
- 2 tablespoons rolled oats
- 3 ice cubes

Directions:

1. Combine the coconut milk, pear, swiss card, cinnamon, rolled oats honey, and green tea into the blender and puree.
2. Add the ice cubes and blend until smooth.
3. Pour in any water for your desired consistency.

Cranberry Quinoa Granola

Prep time: 5 minutes

Cook time: 40 minutes

Serving size: 5

Nutritional information: Calories-116; Carbs-21 grams; Fat-2 grams; Protein-3 grams

Ingredients:

- 1/8 cup pure maple syrup
- 1 cup quinoa flakes
- 1 teaspoons vanilla extract
- ½ cup cranberries (fresh is best)
- 1 teaspoon olive oil

Directions:

1. Set the heat on your oven to 350°F
2. Lay a piece of parchment paper on a cookie sheet.
3. Set a pan on medium heat and combine the maple syrup, cranberries, vanilla, and olive oil. Cook for one minute, or until you start to see bubbles.
4. Turn off the heat and mash the cranberries.
5. Add the flakes into the cranberry mixture and toss together.

6. Spread the granola on the parchment paper.
7. Place in the oven on the middle rack and set the timer for 10 minutes.
8. Remove the pan and toss the granola around.
9. Place the pan back into the oven but on the top rack. Bake for another 25 to 30 minutes or until it's crispy with a light brown color.
10. Remove the pan and allow the granola to cool as it will become crispier.

Almond Butter Hot Cereal Instant Flax Meal

Prep time: 5 to 7 minutes

Cook time: none

Serving size: 1

Nutritional information: Calories-293; Carbs-22 grams; Fat-12 grams; Protein-8 grams

Ingredients:

- 1 tablespoon almond butter
- ¼ cup flaxseed meal
- ¼ teaspoon cinnamon
- ½ cup boiling water
- ½ grapefruit as side

Directions:

1. Combine the boiling water and flaxseed meal into a bowl. Stir well.
2. Mix in the cinnamon and almond butter.
3. Let the hot cereal thicken for one to two minutes.
4. Serve with a side of grapefruit.

Nutty Oatmeal with Blueberries

Prep time: 5 minutes

Cook time: 30 minutes

Serving size: 4

Nutritional information: Calories-246; Carbs-24 grams; Fat-14 grams; Protein-8 grams

Ingredients:

- 1 cup steel-cut oats
- ½ teaspoon ground nutmeg
- 1 cup blueberries
- 3 tablespoons almond butter
- ½ cup whole almonds
- 3 cups water
- 1 teaspoon ground cinnamon
- Ground ginger to taste

Directions:

1. Pour the water into a medium saucepan over medium heat and bring to a boil.
2. Add the oats, stir, and reduce the heat to low. Allow the oats to simmer for about 20 minutes, or until they're tender.
3. Combine the cinnamon, nutmeg, almond butter, and ginger. Mix well and then simmer for another 10 minutes.
4. Divide into bowls and top with whole almonds and blueberries.

Strawberry Breakfast Quinoa

Prep time: 5 minutes

Cook time: 20 minutes

Serving size: 4

Nutritional information: Calories-161; Carbs-22 grams; Fat-5 grams; Protein-5 grams

Ingredients:

- 1 cup unsweetened almond milk
- 2 cups water
- ½ cup quinoa
- 1 teaspoons pure vanilla extract

- ½ cup rolled oats
- 1 cup sliced strawberries (fresh is best)
- Pinch of sea salt

Directions:

1. Place a medium pot over medium-high heat.
2. Bring the almond milk, water, vanilla, quinoa, oats, and salt to a boil while stirring occasionally.
3. Reduce heat and simmer for 20 minutes or until cereal is thick and creamy.
4. Transfer the cereal to a bowl and top with strawberries.

Vegetable Hash

Prep time: 10 minutes

Cook time: 30 minutes

Serving size: 4

Nutritional information: Calories-149; Carbs-12 grams; Fat-8 grams; Protein-9 grams

Ingredients:

- 1 chopped sweet onion
- ½ pound sliced brussel sprouts

- 4 eggs
- 1 chopped bell pepper
- 2 cups sliced mushrooms
- 1 tablespoon olive oil
- 2 tablespoons minced garlic
- 2 teaspoons chopped thyme
- sea salt and black pepper to taste

Directions:

1. Set the temperature of your oven to 400°F
2. Set a burner to medium-high heat and place a skillet on top.
3. Pour in the olive oil and allow it to heat up.
4. Sauté the onions and garlic for 3 to 4 minutes.
5. Combine the mushrooms, brussel sprouts, bell pepper, and thyme. Sauté for another 15 minutes, or until the ingredients are caramelized.
6. Season the vegetables to taste.
7. Make four wells in the mixture and add one egg in each spot.
8. Set the skillet in the oven and bake for 10 minutes or until the eggs are done.

Almond Pancakes

Prep time: 5 minutes

Cook time: 15 minutes

Serving size: 4

Nutritional information: Calories-228; Carbs-6 grams; Fat-20 grams; Protein-10 grams

Ingredients:

- 1 cup unsweetened almond milk
- 2 cups almond flour
- 2 teaspoons baking powder
- 2 tablespoons coconut oil
- 1 tablespoon pure vanilla extract
- 4 eggs
- 1 teaspoons ground nutmeg
- 1 teaspoon ground cinnamon

Directions:

1. In a large bowl combine the nutmeg, cinnamon, baking powder, and almond flour. Whisk well.
2. In a separate bowl whisk the eggs. Then add the almond milk and vanilla. Mix well.
3. Pour the liquid into the dry ingredients mixture. Stir until all ingredients are combined.

4. Set a large skillet on medium heat. Melt 1 tablespoons of coconut oil.
5. Divide the pancake batter into ¼ and pour each into the skillet.
6. Cook for about three minutes and then flip each pancake.
7. Cook for another two minutes or until the pancakes are golden brown.
8. Repeat with the remaining batter and serve with your favorite toppings.

A Simple Low-Carb Breakfast

Prep time: 10 minutes

Cook time: 10 minutes

Serving size: 1

Nutritional information: Calories-434; Carbs-5 grams; Fat-35 grams; Protein-21 grams

Ingredients:

- 4 broccoli sticks
- 2 eggs
- 2 cups water
- 1 tablespoon cream
- 3 slices bacon

- 1 large sliced crimini mushroom
- ¼ sliced avocado
- 1 teaspoon butter
- Pinch of salt and pepper for seasoning

Directions:

1. Pour the water into a saucepan and set on medium-high heat.
2. Add the broccoli sticks and allow to boil for three minutes.
3. Set a frying pan on another burner and turn to medium heat.
4. Place the strips of bacon in the pan and cook until both sides are crispy.
5. Remove the bacon but keep the grease in the pan.
6. Set the broccoli sticks into the grease along with the mushrooms and fry until both are tender.
7. In a bowl whisk the cream and eggs.
8. Pour the eggs into a separate pan or remove the broccoli and mushrooms and scramble the eggs in the bacon grease.
9. Add everything to a plate and serve.

Soup and Salad

Tomato Soup

Prep time: 10 minutes

Cook time: 20 minutes

Serving size: 4

Nutritional information: Calories-146; Carbs-15 grams; Fat-16 grams; Protein-7 grams

Ingredients:

- 4 cups sodium-free chicken broth
- 1 tablespoon olive oil
- 1 tablespoon minced garlic
- 1 chopped small onion
- 48 oz. sodium-free diced tomatoes
- Sea salt and pepper for seasoning

Directions:

1. Put a large saucepan over medium heat and pour in the olive oil.
2. Once the oil is sizzling, sauté the garlic and onions for a few minutes.

3. Pour in the broth, tomatoes, and seasonings. Combine the ingredients thoroughly.
4. Stir occasionally until the soup reaches a boil and then reduce the heat to simmer. Allow it to cook for another 15 minutes.
5. Turn off the heat and transfer the soup into a blender. Cover the blender but use a towel to hold the cover. Pulse until the soup is pureed but remember to release steam every 20 to 30 seconds to release pressure.
6. Return the soup to the saucepan and add the seasonings to taste.

Chicken Minestrone

Prep time: 15 minutes

Cook time: 50 minutes

Serving size: 8

Nutritional information: Calories-101; Carbs-10 grams; Fat-3 grams; Protein-12 grams

Ingredients:

- 1 chopped sweet onion
- 4 chopped celery stalks, keep the greens
- 1 tablespoon olive oil
- 2 cups shredded cabbage

- 6 cups sodium-free chicken stock
- 28 oz sodium-free diced tomatoes
- 4 cups spinach
- 1 tablespoon minced garlic
- 2 cups chopped cooked chicken
- Italian seasoning and sea salt to taste

Directions:

1. In a large stockpot, heat up the olive oil on medium-high.
2. Sauté the onions and garlic until they're soft.
3. Combine the cabbage and celery. Sauté for another 3 to 4 minutes.
4. Mix in the chicken stock and diced tomatoes. Bring the soup to a boil.
5. Reduce the heat to simmer and allow it to cook for another 30 to 35 minutes.
6. Add in the spinach, chicken and seasonings. Cook for 5 more minutes or until the spinach is wilted and chicken is heated thoroughly.
7. Season the soup to your taste before serving.

Spicy Vegetable Soup

Prep time: 25 minutes

Cook time: 45 minutes

Serving size: 4

Nutritional information: Calories-171; Carbs-21 grams; Fat-7 grams; Protein-7 grams

Ingredients:

- ½ chopped fennel bulb
- 2 carrots, cut in half crosswise
- 2 teaspoons olive oil
- 2 teaspoons minced garlic
- 1 chopped onion
- 1 diced sweet potato
- 2 chopped celery stalks
- 2 cups shredded green cabbage
- 8 cups sodium-free chicken broth
- ¼ teaspoon chili powder
- 2 teaspoons chopped thyme (fresh is best)
- 1 cup shredded kale
- Sea salt, red pepper flakes, and ground pepper to taste

Directions:

1. Place a large stockpot on a burner and set it to medium-high heat.
2. Pour in the olive oil and allow it to sizzle.
3. Sauté the garlic, onion, and celery for five minutes.
4. Continue to sauté as you add the carrots, fennel, cabbage, and potato for another five minutes.
5. Stir in the chicken broth and seasonings.
6. Heat the soup until it starts to boil. Reduce the heat to simmer and allow it to cook for another 30 minutes.
7. Add in the kale and simmer for another 4 minutes.

8. Taste the soup and add more seasoning if preferred before serving.

Coconut and Ginger Soup

Prep time: 10 minutes

Cook time: 20 minutes

Serving size: 4

Nutritional information: Calories-372; Carbs-40 grams; Fat-20 grams; Protein-14 grams

Ingredients:

- 1 chopped onion
- 1 tablespoon coconut oil
- 4 chopped celery stalks
- 6 cups sodium-free vegetable stock
- 1 tablespoon ginger
- 1 tablespoon ground cumin
- 2 teaspoons minced garlic
- 15 oz sodium-free navy beans
- 4 cups chopped kale
- 1 cup coconut milk
- Pepper and sea salt to taste

Directions:

1. Place a large stockpot over medium-high heat and add the coconut oil.
2. Once the oil is melted, sauté the onions, garlic, and ginger for 3 to 4 minutes.
3. Continue to sauté as you add in the celery and cumin for another 4 minutes.
4. Combine the olive oil and navy beans. Stir well.
5. Bring the soup to a boil and then reduce the heat to low. Simmer for 10 minutes.
6. Transfer the soup to an immersion blender. Use a towel to hold the cover down and set the blender to pulse. Puree the soup but release the steam every 20 to 30 seconds by stopping the blender and lifting the cover. If you don't do this the steam can make the cover blow off of the blender and you can receive burns.
7. Return the soup to the stockpot and combine the kale, milk, and seasonings.
8. Heat until the kale wilts and taste. Add any more seasonings to your liking.

Citrus Seafood Soup

Prep time: 15 minutes

Cook time: 15 minutes

Serving size: 4

Nutritional information: Calories-215; Carbs-9 grams; Fat-5 grams; Protein-32 grams

Ingredients:

- 6 cups sodium-free vegetable broth
- ½ cup clam juice
- 1 teaspoons olive oil
- 1 teaspoon ginger
- 1 diced carrot
- 2 teaspoons minced garlic
- Zest and juice from 1 lime
- 6 halved sea scallops
- 12 oz. white fish fillets, chop into 1-inch pieces
- 2 thinly sliced scallions, white and green parts only
- 2 tablespoons of cilantro
- 1 diced red bell pepper
- ¼ teaspoon red pepper flakes

Directions:

1. Using a stockpot, set a burner to medium-high heat.
2. Pour in the olive oil and allow it to warm up.

3. Sauté the garlic and ginger until they become soft.
4. Add the clam juice and chicken broth then bring the soup to a boil.
5. Set the heat to low and toss in the scallops, fish, and carrots. Cook for 8 to 10 minutes.
6. Blend the scallions, zest, juice, red pepper flakes, bell pepper, and cilantro. Mix well.
7. Continue to simmer the soup for another one to two minutes before serving.

Turkey and Cauliflower Chowder

Prep time: 10 minutes

Cook time: 30 minutes

Serving size: 8

Nutritional information: Calories-199; Carbs-9 grams; Fat-8 grams; Protein-24 grams

Ingredients:

- 1 tablespoon olive oil
- 1 chopped sweet onion
- 4 cups cooked turkey, white or dark
- 8 cups sodium-free turkey stock, can substitute chicken stock
- 2 teaspoons minced garlic

- ½ head cauliflower chopped into florets
- 1 diced sweet potato
- ½ cup coconut milk
- Your favorite seasonings (sea salt, pepper, paprika, Italian, etc.)

Directions:

1. Put a large stockpot over medium-high heat.
2. Pour in the olive oil and bring to a sizzle.
3. Sauté the garlic and onion for five minutes.
4. Combine the turkey meat, stock, and potato.
5. When the soup begins to point, reduce the heat and allow it to simmer for 20 minutes.
6. Add in the cauliflower and continue to simmer until it becomes tender.
7. Pour in the coconut milk and any seasonings. Stir well.
8. Taste and add in any more seasonings you desire.

Split Pea Soup

Prep time: 10 minutes

Cook time: 2 hours and 30 minutes

Serving size: 4

Nutritional information: Calories-350; Carbs-45 grams; Fat-25 grams; Protein-26 grams

Ingredients:

- 1 ½ cups dried split peas
- 2 teaspoons minced garlic
- 1 tablespoon olive oil
- 1 chopped onion
- 4 chopped celery stalks
- 6 cups sodium free chicken broth, can substitute vegetable stock
- Italian seasoning to taste
- Basil

Directions:

1. Set a large saucepan to medium-high heat.
2. Heat up the olive oil.
3. Sauté the garlic, onions, and celery for five minutes.
4. Pour in the stock and peas.
5. Cook until the soup starts to boil.
6. Reduce heat to low and simmer for about 2 hours, or until the peas are tender.
7. Season the soup to your liking.
8. Top with basil before serving.

Mediterranean Quinoa Salad

Prep time: 20 minutes

Cook time: none

Serving size: 4

Nutritional information: Calories-422; Carbs-37 grams; Fat-39 grams; Protein-8 grams

Ingredients for the salad:

- 2 cups quinoa
- 2 scallions, white and green parts chopped
- ½ diced cucumber
- 2 chopped tomatoes
- 1 cubed red bell pepper
- 1 cubed yellow bell pepper
- 2 tablespoons minced parsley

Ingredients for the vinaigrette:

- 2 tablespoon lemon juice
- 1 teaspoon Dijon mustard
- 2 tablespoon apple cider vinegar
- ½ cup olive oil
- 2 tablespoon chopped oregano
- Pinch of sea salt and black pepper

Directions for the vinaigrette:

1. Combine the lemon juice, vinegar, mustard, and oregano in a bowl. Whisk well.
2. Add in sea salt, pepper, and olive oil until fully incorporated. Set in the fridge while you make the salad.

Directions for the salad:

1. Combine the tomatoes, peppers, quinoa, scallions, and cucumber into a large bowl. Toss gently.
2. Pour the vinaigrette into the bowl.
3. Sprinkle parsley and toss the salad before serving.

Bean and Fruit Salad

Prep time: 15 minutes

Cook time: none

Serving size: 4

Nutritional information: Calories-195; Carbs-36 grams; Fat-2 grams; Protein-11 grams

Ingredients:

- 1 cup dried and rinsed navy beans
- 1 cup dried and rinsed red kidney beans
- 1 cup dried and rinsed chickpeas
- 2 cups green beans
- ¼ cup shredded cilantro
- 1 pitted, chopped peach
- 2 tablespoons lime juice
- 1 scallion with chopped green and white parts
- ½ diced red bell pepper
- Pepper, sea salt, and parsley for seasoning

Directions:

1. Cut the green beans into 1-inch slices and blanch until tender.
2. In a large bowl combine all of the ingredients except for the seasonings and gently stir.

3. Add in the seasonings to your taste. Toss the salad before serving.

Coleslaw

Prep time: 30 minutes with 2 hours marinating time

Cook time: none

Serving size: 4

Nutritional information: Calories-151; Carbs-12 grams; Fat-10 grams; Protein-5 grams

Ingredients for the salad:

- 1 shredded carrot
- ½ head cabbage, shredded
- 2 cups french cut snow peas
- 2 diced shallots
- ¼ cup slivered almonds
- 2 french cut daikon radishes
- 2 tablespoons cilantro

Ingredients for the dressing:

- 2 tablespoons sesame oil
- 1 tablespoon lime juice
- 1 teaspoon grated ginger
- 2 tablespoons rice vinegar

- 1 teaspoon orange zest
- ½ teaspoon minced garlic

Directions for the dressing:

1. Combine all of the ingredients and mix well. Set aside.

Directions for the salad:

1. In a large bowl, combine all of the ingredients and toss together.
2. Pour the dressing over the salad and toss until all the ingredients are well coated.
3. To get the best flavor, set in the fridge to marinate for 2 hours before serving.

Thai Tahini Slaw

Prep time: 20 minutes

Cook time: none

Serving size: 4

Nutritional information: Calories-247; Carbs-19 grams; Fat-16 grams; Protein-9 grams

Ingredients:

- 2 shredded carrots
- 1 shredded head of cabbage

- ½ cup chopped roasted peanuts
- ½ cup tahini peanut sauce
- 1 scallion, white and green parts chopped
- 2 tablespoons shredded cilantro

Directions:

1. Combine the carrots, cabbage, roasted peanuts, and scallions. Stir gently.
2. Pour the sauce and cilantro on the salad and toss well before serving.

Pecan Spinach Salad

Prep time: 10 minutes

Cook time: none

Serving size: 4

Nutritional information: Calories-382; Carbs-24 grams; Fat-24 grams; Protein-9 grams

Ingredients:

- 4 hard boiled eggs cut into eighths
- ½ cup chopped pecans
- 8 cups baby spinach
- 1 cored and diced pear

- Your favorite dressing, such as poppy seed or vinaigrette

Directions:

1. Divide the spinach, eggs, and pear onto four plates.
2. Drizzle your dressing over the top.
3. Sprinkle with pecans and serve.

Wild Rice Peach Salad

Prep time: 15 minutes

Cook time: none

Serving size: 4

Nutritional information: Calories-215; Carbs-23 grams; Fat-13 grams; Protein-5 grams

Ingredients:

- 1 diced red bell pepper
- 4 cups shredded kale
- 2 pitted and diced peaches
- ½ cup cooked wild rice
- ½ cup balsamic or raspberry dressing
- 2 tablespoons slivered almonds

Directions:

1. In a large bowl toss all of the ingredients but the slivered almonds.
2. Before serving, sprinkle with the almonds.

Salmon-Arugula Salad

Prep time: 10 minutes

Cook time: none

Serving size: 4

Nutritional information: Calories-219; Carbs-5 grams; Fat-11 grams; Protein-22 grams

Ingredients:

- 1 cup shredded fennel
- 8 cups baby arugula
- 8 sliced radishes
- 20 oz. cooked salmon fillets
- ½ cup vinaigrette

Directions:

1. In a bowl, toss all of the ingredients except the salmon.
2. Divide the salad onto four plates and top with salmon before serving.

Snacks and Sides

Zucchini Fries

Prep time: 15 minutes

Cook time: 20 minutes

Serving size: 4

Nutritional information: Calories-197; Carbs-20 grams; Fat-9 grams; Protein-7 grams

Ingredients:

- ½ cup cornstarch
- 1 pound zucchini
- 2 cups almond flour
- 2 eggs
- 1 teaspoon garlic powder
- Sea salt and pepper for seasoning

Directions:

1. Preheat your oven to 400°F
2. Line a baking pan with parchment paper.
3. Cut the zucchini into a ½-inch wide and 4-inch long pieces.

4. In a small bowl, add the cornstarch.
5. In a separate small bowl, whisk the eggs.
6. In a third small bowl combine garlic powder and almond flour.
7. Take one of the zucchini slices and roll it in the cornstarch, then eggs, and finally flour mixture. Set the vegetable on the pan and then repeat the process with the remaining pieces.
8. Season the fries and bake for 20 minutes or until desired crispness.

Creamed Spinach and Leeks

Prep time: 10 minutes

Cook time: 20 minutes

Serving size: 4

Nutritional information: Calories-148; Carbs-12 grams; Fat-11 grams; Protein-3 grams

Ingredients:

- 3 leeks, green and white parts cleaned and sliced
- 4 cups spinach
- ½ teaspoon ground nutmeg
- ¼ cup sodium-free chicken stock
- 1 tablespoon olive oil

- ½ cup coconut milk
- Sea salt and pepper for seasoning

Directions:

1. Set a large skillet over medium heat and let the olive oil sizzle.
2. Sauté the leeks for 10 minutes or until they're tender and caramelized.
3. Add in the spinach and sauté for 4 to 5 minutes or until it's welted.
4. Pour in the chicken stock and coconut milk. Stir continuously as it cooks for 4 minutes.
5. Season the cream with nutmeg, pepper, and salt before serving.

Spring Vegetable Medley

Prep time: 15 minutes

Cook time: 15 minutes

Serving size: 4

Nutritional information: Calories-90; Carbs-13 grams; Fat-4 grams; Protein-3 grams

Ingredients:

- 1 teaspoon minced garlic

- ½ head broccoli, cut into florets
- ½ head cauliflower, cut into florets
- 1 tablespoon olive oil
- 2 sliced carrots
- 1 red bell pepper, sliced into strips
- 1 cup green beans, chopped into 1-inch pieces
- 1 yellow zucchini, sliced into thin round pieces
- Thyme and pepper for seasoning

Directions:

1. With a large skillet over medium-high heat, pour in the olive oil.
2. Sauté the garlic for two minutes or until it's softened.
3. Toss in the carrots and sauté for three minutes.
4. Sauté the broccoli and cauliflower in the mixture for four minutes.
5. Add the rest of the vegetables and sauté for another five minutes or until they're all crisp.
6. Sprinkle the medley with thyme and pepper before serving.

Crispy Onion Rings

Prep time: 20 minutes

Cook time: 20 minutes

Serving size: 4

Nutritional information: Calories-220; Carbs-32 grams; Fat-8 grams; Protein-7 grams

Ingredients:

- Cooking spray
- 2 tablespoons arrowroot flour
- 1 cup sodium-free vegetable stock
- 1 ½ cups flour blend, gluten-free
- 2 large onions, cut into ½-inch thick slices
- 2 cups almond flour

Directions:

1. Turn the temperature of your oven to 425°F
2. Spray a cooking sheet.
3. Combine the flour blend, arrowroot flour, and vegetable stock in a large bowl. Whisk until it has a smooth consistency.
4. In a separate bowl pour in the almond flour.
5. Separate the onions into individual rings and choose the 40 best ones.
6. Dip the onions into the batter. Ensure they're coated well and then dip them into the almond flour.
7. Set the coated onion on the baking sheet. Repeat the process with the rest of the rings.
8. Lightly spray the onions with cooking spray and set in the oven.
9. Flip the onion rings at the halfway mark.
10. Remove from the oven when they're at your desired crispiness and enjoy.

Spice-Roasted Chickpeas

Prep time: 10 minutes

Cook time: 45 minutes

Serving size: 4

Nutritional information: Calories-154; Carbs-22 grams; Fat-4 grams; Protein-7 grams

Ingredients:

- 2 tablespoons olive oil
- 2 cups drained and rinsed sodium-free chickpeas
- ¼ teaspoon ground cumin
- ½ teaspoon ground turmeric

Directions:

1. Preheat your oven to 375°F
2. Combine the olive oil, chickpeas, turmeric, and cumin in a large bowl. Mix well.
3. Spread the mixture over a baking sheet evenly. You can use parchment paper to keep the food from sticking to the pan.
4. Place in your oven and set the timer to 45 minutes.
5. Cool the chickpeas and transfer them into an airtight container. They can sit at room temperature for five days.

Sweet Potato Hummus

Prep time: 15 minutes

Cook time: none

Serving size: 4

Nutritional information: Calories-251; Carbs-25 grams; Fat-15 grams; Protein-6 grams

Ingredients:

- ½ cup rinsed and drained chickpeas
- 1 ½ cups cook sweet potato, mashed
- 2 tablespoons olive oil
- ¼ cup tahini
- ¼ teaspoon ground coriander
- ¼ teaspoon ground cumin
- 1 teaspoon minced garlic

Directions:

1. In a blinder, add the chickpeas, sweet potato, olive oil, tahini, garlic, coriander, and cumin. Puree for a smooth consistency.
2. Transfer the hummus into an airtight container. You can keep it in the fridge for up to seven days.

Oat Energy Balls

Prep time: 10 minutes plus 30 minutes to chill

Cook time: none

Serving size: makes a dozen balls

Nutritional information: Calories-181; Carbs-23 grams; Fat-8 grams; Protein-6 grams

Ingredients:

- ½ cup sunflower seeds
- 2 cups rolled oats
- ¼ cup dried blueberries
- ¼ cup almond butter
- ¼ teaspoon nutmeg
- 2 tablespoons of raw honey
- ½ teaspoon cinnamon

Directions:

1. Tear off a piece of parchment paper to line the baking pan.
2. Combine all of the ingredients into a large bowl. Mix well.
3. Roll the ingredients into 1-inch balls and place on the pan.
4. Cover the pan and set it in the fridge for 30 minutes or until the balls become firm.

Nutmeg Pear Chips

Prep time: 10 minutes

Cook time: 45 minutes

Serving size: 4

Nutritional information: Calories-86; Carbs-23 grams; Fat-0 grams; Protein-1 gram

Ingredients:

- 1 teaspoon nutmeg
- 4 peeled, cored, and thinly sliced pears
- Salt to taste

Directions:

1. Set your oven to 300°F
2. Cover a baking sheet with parchment paper.
3. Layer the pears onto the paper so they don't overlap.
4. Sprinkle with salt.
5. Place in the oven for 45 minutes or until the chips are crispy and brown.
6. Cool them completely. Store them in an airtight container at room temperature for up to five days.

Dill Carrot Ribbons

Prep time: 15 minutes

Cook time: 5 minutes

Serving size: 4

Nutritional information: Calories-79; Carbs-16 grams; Fat-2 grams; Protein-2 grams

Ingredients:

- ½ pound carrots peeled and sliced into ribbons. Tip: using a vegetable peeler is easiest.
- 1 teaspoon olive oil
- 1 tablespoon chopped dill, fresh is best
- 1 tablespoon lemon juice
- A pinch of sea salt

Directions:

1. Heat up the olive oil by pouring it into a skillet over medium-high temperature.
2. Sauté the carrot ribbons for five minutes. Carefully stir them around until they become crispy.
3. Pour the lemon juice and dill in a bowl.
4. Transfer the carrots into the bowl and add seasoning to taste.
5. Gently toss ingredients before serving.

Sweet Potato Salad

Prep time: 5 minutes, plus 10 to 15 minutes to cool

Cook time: 30 minutes

Serving size: 4

Nutritional information: Calories-255; Carbs-35 grams; Fat-10 grams; Protein-3 grams

Ingredients for the salad:

- 1 ½ pounds sweet potato, peeled and cut into 1-inch pieces
- 1 scallion, green and white pieces chopped only
- 1 tablespoon olive oil
- ¼ teaspoon celery salt
- ¼ teaspoon paprika

Ingredients for the dressing:

- ¼ cup apple cider vinegar
- 1 teaspoon chopped or dried thyme leaves
- 1 tablespoon raw honey
- 2 tablespoons olive oil

Directions to make the dressing:

1. Whisk together all of the dressing ingredients in a small bowl. Set aside.

Directions to make the salad:

1. Preheat your oven to 400°F
2. Layer the potato chunks on a baking sheet.
3. Drizzle with olive oil.
4. Place in the oven and bake for 30 minutes or until they're caramelized.
5. After the potatoes cool for 10 minutes, transfer them into a bowl.
6. Add the scallions and pour the dressing over the salad. Toss the mixture to coat the potatoes completely.
7. Season to your taste buds' desire.

Bean Cannellini Pilaf

Prep time: 10 minutes

Cook time: 15 minutes

Serving size: 4

Nutritional information: Calories-173; Carbs-25 grams; Fat-4 grams; Protein-10 grams

Ingredients:

- 2 chopped celery stalks
- 1 chopped carrot
- 1 chopped onion

- 1 tablespoon olive oil
- 1 teaspoon ground cumin
- 1 teaspoon minced garlic
- 2 cups cannellini beans, drained and rinsed
- 2 tablespoons chopped parsley leaves
- ½ cup edamame
- 1 tablespoon chopped oregano leaves

Directions:

1. Heat up the olive oil in a large skillet.
2. Sauté the carrot, celery, garlic, and onions for 5 to 7 minutes or until they're soft and caramelized.
3. Combine the edamame, beans, and cumin and cook for another 5 minutes.
4. Sprinkle with parsley and oregano before serving.

Tomato and Spinach Stuffed Mushrooms

Prep time: 10 minutes

Cook time: 20 minutes

Serving size: 4

Nutritional information: Calories-50; Carbs-5 grams; Fat-3 grams; Protein-3 grams

Ingredients:

- 16 large white mushrooms, de-stemmed
- ½ cup chopped tomato
- 1 cup chopped spinach
- 2 teaspoons olive oil, divided
- 1 chopped scallion, white and green parts only
- 2 teaspoons minced garlic
- Cayenne pepper for seasoning, can substitute black pepper

Directions:

1. Turn your oven to 375°F
2. Line a baking sheet with aluminum foil and set the mushrooms down.
3. Drizzle with one teaspoon olive oil and set in the oven for five minutes.
4. Add the other teaspoon of olive oil to a large skillet on medium heat.
5. Sauté the garlic for three minutes or until softened.
6. Combine the scallion, spinach, and tomato in the pan and sauté for another four minutes.
7. Season the filling with cayenne pepper.
8. Scoop the filling into the mushrooms and set in the oven for another five minutes.

Roasted Vegetables

Prep time: 15 minutes

Cook time: 15 minutes

Serving size: 6

Nutritional information: Calories-92; Carbs-11 grams; Fat-5 grams; Protein-3 grams

Ingredients:

- 2 cups broccoli florets
- 1 cup chopped butternut squash
- 2 tablespoons olive oil, plus extra for grease
- 2 cups chopped green beans, 2-inch pieces
- 2 cups button mushrooms
- 1 diced yellow summer squash
- 1 zucchini
- 1 diced onion
- 1 diced red bell pepper
- 4 minced garlic cloves
- 2 tablespoons balsamic vinegar
- 1 ½ teaspoon dried thyme
- 1 teaspoon dried oregano
- 1 teaspoon rosemary

Directions:

1. Set the temperature of your oven to 425°F

2. Grease a baking sheet with olive oil.
3. Cut the zucchini in quarters lengthwise and then 2-inch pieces.
4. In a bowl, mix the broccoli, zucchini, beans, mushrooms, summer squash, butternut squash, red onion and bell pepper. Gently stir.
5. Spread the mixture on the baking sheet.
6. Drizzle two tablespoons of olive oil and vinegar over the vegetables.
7. Sprinkle the rosemary, thyme, and oregano on the mixture. Toss gently to combine the ingredients.
8. Set in the oven and bake for 13 to 15 minutes or until the vegetables are tender.

Brussel Sprouts with Berries and Nuts

Prep time: 15 minutes

Cook time: 10 minutes

Serving size: 8

Nutritional information: Calories-113; Carbs-12 grams; Fat-7 grams; Protein-4 grams

Ingredients:

- 2 teaspoons olive oil, divided
- 1 pound trimmed brussel sprouts

- ⅓ cup shelled and chopped pistachios
- ½ diced red onion
- ½ cup cranberries, fresh or frozen
- 1 tablespoon hemp seeds
- Salt and pepper for seasoning

Directions:

1. Slice each brussel sprout in half through the stem. Then, chop into thin slices.
2. In a large skillet bring one teaspoon of olive oil to a sizzle and sauté the onions for five minutes.
3. Pour in the remaining olive oil with the brussel sprouts and cook until they become tender.
4. Add in the cranberries, pistachios, seeds, and seasoning. Stir well before serving.

Vegetarian

Crispy Almond Tofu

Prep time: 30 minutes

Cook time: 25 minutes

Serving size: 4

Nutritional information: Calories-104; Carbs-3 grams; Fat-5 grams; Protein-11 grams

Ingredients:

- 1 cup almond meal
- 2 egg whites
- ½ teaspoon paprika
- 16 oz. tofu, cut into 12 squares
- ½ teaspoon garlic powder

Directions:

1. Lay a piece of parchment paper over a baking sheet.
2. Whisk the eggs in a small bowl.
3. In a different bowl, whisk the almond meal, garlic powder, and paprika.
4. Dip each piece of tofu into the egg whites and then the separate bowl. Ensure they are fully coated before placing them on the baking sheet.
5. Cover the tofu and let it sit in the fridge for 20 minutes.
6. Preheat the oven to 375°F
7. Transfer the baking sheet into the oven and set the timer for 25 minutes or until they're golden crispy.

Kale and Tofu Scramble

Prep time: 5 minutes

Cook time: 15 minutes

Serving size: 4

Nutritional information: Calories-207; Carbs-14 grams; Fat-13 grams; Protein-14 grams

Ingredients:

- ¼ cup nutritional yeast
- 1 teaspoon paprika
- 15 oz. tofu
- 1 teaspoon ground turmeric
- 2 teaspoons olive oil
- 2 cups de-stemmed and chopped kale
- 1 teaspoon garlic powder
- 1 diced avocado
- ¼ cup chopped onion
- ½ cup halved cherry tomatoes

Directions:

1. Drain the tofu and cut them into strips. Set the tofu on a plate with paper towels surrounding them. Put a small weight on top of the tofu so they can continue to drain.

2. Pour olive oil into a large skillet and set on medium heat.
3. Add the tofu and break them into smaller pieces.
4. Combine the yeast, turmeric, paprika, and garlic powder into a bowl. Sprinkle over the tofu and toss to mix.
5. Stir in the tomatoes, kale, and onions. Cook for 10 minutes while stirring occasionally.
6. Mix in the avocado and serve.

Grilled Cauliflower Steaks with Black Bean Salsa

Prep time: 10 minutes

Cook time: 8 minutes

Serving size: 4

Nutritional information: Calories-674; Carbs-56 grams; Fat-13 grams; Protein-15 grams

Ingredients:

- 2 tablespoons extra virgin olive oil
- 1 head of cauliflower
- ½ cup chopped cherry tomatoes
- ¼ cup minced cilantro
- 2 cups chopped mango
- ½ teaspoon ground cumin

- Juice from 2 limes
- 1 teaspoon chili powder
- 1 sliced avocado
- ½ teaspoon paprika
- 15 oz. drained and rinsed black beans
- 2 chopped onions

Directions:

1. Remove the head and the outer leaves of the cauliflower.
2. Starting from the middle, cut four 1-inch thick steaks horizontally.
3. Place a grill pan over medium heat.
4. Brush each side of the steaks with olive oil.
5. Grill each side for four to five minutes.
6. To start making the salsa, add the cherry tomatoes into a bowl.
7. Combine the cumin, paprika, chili powder, mango, beans, green onion, cilantro, and lemon juice. Mix well.
8. To serve, set a steak on a plate, add a few pieces of avocado, and top with salsa.

Split Pea Falafel

Prep time: 10 minutes

Cook time: 50 minutes

Serving size: 4

Nutritional information: Calories-127; Carbs-19 grams; Fat-3 grams; Protein-7 grams

Ingredients:

- ½ cup dried split peas
- ⅓ cup chopped onion
- 2 cups water
- 4 garlic cloves
- 1 teaspoon ground cumin
- ½ cup parsley leaves
- ½ teaspoon salt
- 1 teaspoon coriander
- 2 teaspoons olive oil plus more for brushing
- ½ teaspoon black pepper
- 2 tablespoons chickpea flour

Directions:

1. Set the temperature of your oven to 400°F
2. Wash and drain the peas in a colander.
3. Place a medium saucepan to medium-high heat.

4. Add the water and peas, cook until the peas are tender and water boils.
5. Drain the peas and let them cool for a couple of minutes.
6. In a blender, combine the peas, parsley, onion, salt, cumin, garlic, pepper, coriander, and olive oil. Press pulse until the mixture is coarse.
7. Transfer the mixture into a bowl.
8. Add the chickpea flour and merge all ingredients together. If the dough is too sticky, sprinkle more flour and mix.
9. Line parchment paper over a baking pan.
10. Rubs your hands with olive oil and make 1 ½-inch balls out of the dough.
11. Line them onto the pan and brush with more olive oil.
12. Place in the oven for 30 minutes or until the dough is crisp. Serve immediately.

Cauliflower Fried Rice

Prep time: 10 minutes

Cook time: 10 minutes

Serving size: 4

Nutritional information: Calories-195; Carbs-21 grams; Fat-9 grams; Protein-10 grams

Ingredients:

- 5 cups cauliflower florets, about 24 oz.
- 1 tablespoon sesame oil
- ¼ teaspoon white pepper
- 2 tablespoons Bragg's liquid aminos
- 1 tablespoon minced ginger
- 1 cup snow peas
- 2 beaten eggs
- 3 tablespoons olive oil
- 2 minced garlic cloves
- ½ cup bite-size broccoli florets
- 1 diced onion
- 1 diced red bell pepper
- 1 peeled and grated carrots
- 1 teaspoon sesame seeds
- 2 thinly sliced green onions

Directions:

1. To make the cauliflower rice, out the florets in a food processor and pulse for three minutes or until it resembles rice.
2. In a bowl, mix the aminos, ginger, sesame oil, and white pepper. Set aside.
3. Pour two teaspoons of olive oil into a skillet and set to a low setting.
4. Swirl the oil in the pan so the bottom becomes coated.
5. Pour in the eggs and cook for two to three minutes on each side. Only flip once and then chop into pieces once cooked. Transfer onto a plate.

6. Turn the heat to medium-high and add the rest of the olive oil. Cook the onions and garlic until translucent or about three to four minutes.
7. Combine the bell pepper, snow peas, carrots, and broccoli. Cook for three to four minutes or until vegetables are tender.
8. Add in the amino mixture, eggs, cauliflower, and green onions. Stir constantly as it cooks for five minutes.
9. Garnish with sesame seeds before serving.

Southwestern Quinoa Skillet

Prep time: 10 minutes

Cook time: 20 minutes

Serving size: 5

Nutritional information: Calories-231; Carbs-35 grams; Fat-6 grams; Protein-11 grams

Ingredients:

- ½ minced jalapeno
- 2 teaspoons olive oil
- 1 teaspoon ground cumin
- 2 teaspoons garlic powder
- 2 cups cooked quinoa
- ½ teaspoon chili powder

- 1 cup edamame
- 1 cup drained and rinsed sodium-free black beans
- Juice from 1 lime
- 1 cup diced tomato

Directions:

1. Heat the olive oil in a large skillet set to medium-high.
2. Sauté the jalapeno, cumin, garlic, and chili powder for three minutes.
3. Combine the black beans, quinoa, edamame, and tomato. Mix well and cook for 15 minutes.
4. Drizzle the lime juice over the dish before you serve.

Stuffed Mint Eggplant

Prep time: 10 minutes

Cook time: 20 to 25 minutes

Serving size: 4

Nutritional information: Calories-194; Carbs-29 grams; Fat-6 grams; Protein-6 grams

Ingredients:

- 1 tablespoon olive oil
- 2 teaspoons minced garlic
- 2 diced tomatoes

- 2 cups cooked millet
- ½ diced onion
- ½ cup pumpkin seeds
- 1 cup shredded spinach
- 1 tablespoon lemon juice
- 1 tablespoon dried or freshly chopped basil leaves
- ½ teaspoon coriander
- 2 small eggplants

Directions:

1. Cut the eggplants in half and flesh scooped out within a half inch of the skin. You can reserve the flesh for another use, such as making pasta.
2. Turn your oven to 400°F
3. Pour the olive oil into a skillet and set to medium heat. Let the oil warm up.
4. Sauté the onion and garlic for three minutes.
5. Add the rest of the ingredients but the egg plants. Stir until the mixture if fully incorporated.
6. Line a baking sheet with parchment paper.
7. Scoop the mixture into the eggplants and place them on the pan.
8. Set them in the oven until the eggplant is tender, about 20 minutes.
9. You can add a little salt and pepper for extra seasoning before serving.

Vegetable Pecan Burgers

Prep time: 10 minutes plus 30 minutes to chill

Cook time: 15 minutes

Serving size: 4

Nutritional information: Calories-146; Carbs-14 grams; Fat-9 grams; Protein-5 grams

Ingredients:

- 1 can rinsed and drained chickpeas
- 2 teaspoons olive oil, divided
- 1 cup chopped pecans
- ½ diced onion
- 2 teaspoons low-sodium tamari sauce
- 1 teaspoon minced garlic
- ¼ cup cilantro leaves
- ¼ teaspoon ground cinnamon
- ½ teaspoon ground cumin

Directions:

1. Heat one tablespoon olive oil in a skillet over medium temperature.
2. Sauté the garlic and onions until they're lightly caramelized, about five minutes.

3. Transfer the mixture into a food processor. Combine the rest of the ingredients and then pulse until you get a sticky and chopped texture.
4. Divide the mixture into four burgers that are 3 ½ inches in diameter.
5. Set the burgers on a plate, cover, and then set in the fridge for 30 minutes.
6. Line a piece of parchment paper on a baking pan.
7. Set your oven to broil.
8. Take the remaining olive oil and brush the burgers on both sides.
9. Broil the burgers for five minutes on each side.
10. Top with your favorite condiments and serve.

Bean Stuffed Zucchini

Prep time: 10 minutes

Cook time: 25 minutes

Serving size: 4

Nutritional information: Calories-306; Carbs-34 grams; Fat-12 grams; Protein-11 grams

Ingredients:

- 4 zucchini
- ½ diced onion

- 1 cup shredded spinach
- ¼ cup chopped hazelnuts
- 2 tablespoons olive oil, divided
- 2 teaspoons crushed garlic
- 1 grated carrot
- ½ cup millet, cooked
- 2 cups rinsed, drained, and cooked navy beans
- Sea salt and pepper for seasoning

Directions:

1. Set the temperature of your oven to 400°F
2. Place parchment paper on a baking sheet.
3. Cut the zucchinis lengthwise in half and scoop out the seeds. Set the vegetables on the paper.
4. Brush the cut sides with one tablespoon olive oil.
5. Put the zucchini in the oven for six minutes or until soft.
6. Pour the rest of the oil into a skillet over medium-low heat.
7. Sauté the garlic and onions until they're caramelized or for five minutes.
8. Combine the spinach, navy beans, carrot, millet, and hazelnut. Stir well.
9. Once the zucchini is done, remove from the oven and scoop the skillet mix into the vegetable.
10. Set the pan back into the oven for 10 minutes.
11. Season before serving.

Mixed Vegetable Lettuce Wraps

Prep time: 20 minutes

Cook time: 7 minutes

Serving size: 4

Nutritional information: Calories-198; Carbs-24 grams; Fat-8 grams; Protein-9 grams

Ingredients:

- 1 tablespoon coconut oil
- 1 teaspoon crushed garlic
- 1 shredded yellow zucchini
- 8 large Boston lettuce leaves
- 1 shredded carrot
- 1 tablespoon chopped cilantro
- Juice and zest from 1 lime
- ½ cup green beans, cut into ½-inch pieces
- ½ chopped onion
- 1 cup sodium-free red lentils

Directions:

1. Add the oil to a large skillet on medium-high heat.
2. For three minutes, sauté the garlic and onions.
3. Combine the zucchini, green beans, and carrot and continue to sauté for four minutes.

4. Add in the lemon juice, zest, cilantro, and lentils. Stir well.
5. Scoop the filling into the lettuce leaves.
6. Drizzle with olive oil or sprinkle with your favorite seasoning for added visual pleasure and taste before serving.

Southwest Sweet Potatoes

Prep time: 10 minutes

Cook time: 30 minutes

Serving size: 4

Nutritional information: Calories-347; Carbs-50 grams; Fat-10 grams; Protein-13 grams

Ingredients:

- 4 sweet potatoes
- 2 cups sodium-free lentils, cooked
- 1 tablespoon olive oil
- 1 diced avocado
- 2 tablespoons chopped cilantro
- 1 cup salsa
- Seasonings to taste, such as sea salt, pepper, oregano

Directions:

1. Set the temperature of your oven to 400°F
2. Place aluminum foil over a baking sheet.
3. Cut the sweet potatoes into quarters.
4. Add the potatoes and oil into a bowl and toss until well coated.
5. Spread the potatoes over the foil.
6. Sprinkle with your favorite seasonings.
7. Place in the oven and set the timer for 30 minutes.
8. When the potatoes are almost done, pour the salsa and lentils into a skillet over medium heat. Stir constantly until the ingredients are heated through. Turn off the heat and set aside until the potatoes are done.
9. Transfer the potatoes on a plate and add the salsa mixture on top.
10. Add avocado slices on the side and top with cilantro before serving.

Spicy Falafel

Prep time: 20 minutes

Cook time: 10 minutes

Serving size: 4

Nutritional information: Calories-298; Carbs-39 grams; Fat-11 grams; Protein-13 grams

Ingredients:

- ¼ cup almond flour
- 1 diced scallion
- 1 ½ cups sodium-free chickpeas
- 1 egg
- ½ teaspoon ground cumin
- 1 tablespoon olive oil
- 1 chopped tomato
- ½ cup plain low-fat Greek yogurt
- 2 sprouted grain pitas, 6-inches each
- ½ chopped avocado

Directions:

1. Pulse the chickpeas in a blender until they are mashed.
2. Combine the scallion, almond flour, and cumin. Pulse to mix.
3. Add the egg and pulse until the mixture starts sticking together. If you find the texture is too crumbly, add a little water.
4. Divide the mixture into four ½-inch thick patties.
5. Pour the olive oil into a skillet and place on medium heat.
6. Cook the patties for five minutes per side.
7. Remove the patties from the skillet and pat any excess oil off of them.
8. Stuff one pattie into each pita half.
9. Top the falafel with yogurt, tomato, and avocado before serving.

Farmer's Market Paella

Prep time: 15 minutes

Cook time: 25 minutes

Serving size: 4

Nutritional information: Calories-229; Carbs-35 grams; Fat-6 grams; Protein-9 grams

Ingredients:

- 1 cut up red bell pepper
- 1 cup cauliflower florets
- 1 tablespoon olive oil
- 1 chopped onion
- 1 diced zucchini
- 1 thinly sliced carrot
- 2 teaspoons minced garlic
- 2 cups cooked quinoa
- 3 tablespoons chopped parsley

Directions:

1. Pour the olive oil into a skillet and set to medium heat.
2. Sauté garlic and onions for three minutes.
3. Combine the carrots, cauliflower, bell pepper, and zucchini. Sauté for another 10 minutes or until vegetables are crisp.

4. Add the quinoa into the mix and continue to sauté for another 10 minutes.
5. Top with parsley before serving.

Chilled Asian Vegetable Noodles

Prep time: 15 minutes

Cook time: 6 minutes

Serving size: 2

Nutritional information: Calories-296; Carbs-37 grams; Fat-17 grams; Protein-9 grams

Ingredients for the noodles:

- 2 spiralized zucchini or cut ribbons with a vegetable peeler
- 1 cup bean sprouts
- 1 spiralized carrot or cut ribbons with a vegetable peeler
- 1 red bell pepper, julienned
- 1 tablespoon sesame seeds

Ingredients for the sauce

- ¼ cup rice vinegar
- 2 tablespoons coconut aminos
- 1 tablespoon olive oil

- 1 teaspoon raw honey
- 2 teaspoons grated ginger
- 1 teaspoon crushed garlic

Directions for the sauce:

1. In a bowl, combine all of the ingredients. Whisk well and set aside.

Directions for the noodles:

1. Pour the sauce into a skillet on medium heat.
2. Sauté the zucchini, bean sprouts, bell pepper, and carrots for five minutes or until the vegetables become crisp.
3. Top with sesame seeds before serving.

Vegetarian Egg Pizza

Prep time: 20 minutes

Cook time: 40 minutes

Serving size: 4

Nutritional information: Calories-132; Carbs-10 grams; Fat-7 grams; Protein-10 grams

Ingredients:

- ½ cup arugula, divided

- 1 teaspoon chopped thyme
- 2 teaspoons olive oil, divided
- 1 seeded and diced yellow bell pepper
- 1 seeded and diced red bell pepper
- 1 chopped zucchini
- 1 minced onion
- ½ cup sun-dried tomatoes
- 1 cup oyster mushrooms
- 1 tablespoon Dijon mustard
- 3 egg whites
- 3 eggs

Directions:

1. Set the temperature of your oven to 375°F
2. Tear a piece of parchment paper to cover a baking sheet.
3. In a bowl, combine one teaspoon of oil, onion, bell peppers, tomatoes, mushrooms, and zucchini. Toss well.
4. Spread the vegetable mixture on the parchment paper and roast them in the oven for 25 minutes. Remove them and set aside.
5. In a bowl, whisk together the Dijon mustard, eggs, egg whites, and thyme.
6. Pour ½ of the remaining oil into a skillet over medium heat.
7. Add half of the egg mixture and swirl so it's even in the pan.

8. Once the eggs are cooked through, about five minutes, remove them from the skillet.
9. Scoop half of the vegetable mixture on top of the eggs and add half of the arugula.
10. Cut the pizza and keep it warm.
11. Repeat steps six through nine with the remaining ingredients. Cut the second pizza before serving.

Southwestern Rice

Prep time: 20 minutes

Cook time: 45 minutes

Serving size: 6

Nutritional information: Calories-162; Carbs-29 grams; Fat-3 grams; Protein-4 grams

Ingredients:

- 1 chopped green bell pepper
- 1 chopped red bell pepper
- 1 tablespoon olive oil
- 1 teaspoon minced garlic
- ½ finely chopped onion
- 1 finely chopped carrot
- 1 teaspoon ground coriander
- 1 teaspoon ground cumin

- ½ teaspoon ground turmeric
- 2 cups low-sodium chicken broth
- 1 cup brown rice

Directions:

1. Pour the olive oil into a medium saucepan and set on medium heat.
2. Sauté the onions and garlic until caramelized or three to four minutes.
3. Add the cumin, peppers, coriander, turmeric, and carrots. Sauté for another five minutes.
4. Pour in the chicken broth and brown rice. Stir well.
5. Once the rice starts to boil, reduce the heat to simmer and cook for 35 minutes or until all liquid is absorbed. Stir before serving.

Poultry and Meat

Chicken with Ginger Rice Noodles

Prep time: 20 minutes plus 1 hour of soaking time

Cook time: 15 minutes

Serving size: 4

Nutritional information: Calories-554; Carbs-25 grams; Fat-35 grams; Protein-29 grams

Ingredients:

- 1 finely chopped scallion
- 2 tablespoons olive oil
- 4 ounces dried rice noodles
- 2 teaspoons minced garlic
- 2 teaspoons grated ginger
- 2 cups coconut milk
- Zest and juice from 1 lime
- 10 oz. cooked chicken breast, cut into bite-size pieces
- 2 tablespoons chopped cilantro
- 1 cup low-sodium chicken broth
- 2 shredded carrots
- 3 tablespoons chopped peanuts
- 2 cups julienned snow peas

Directions:

1. Combine water and rice noodles in a bowl. You want to ensure the water covers the noodles by about 2 inches. Let it sit for one hour.
2. Pour the oil into a skillet and heat on medium-high.
3. Sauté the ginger, garlic, and scallion for four minutes.
4. Add in the cilantro, coconut milk, lime juice, and lime zest. Stir well.
5. Once the sauce starts to boil, add in the snow peas, chicken, rice noodles, and carrots. Turn the heat down to simmer and let the mixture cook for seven minutes.

6. Top with peanuts and serve.

Breaded Chicken with Mustard

Prep time: 20 minutes

Cook time: 10 minutes

Serving size: 4

Nutritional information: Calories-293; Carbs-1 grams; Fat-17 grams; Protein-33 grams

Ingredients:

- 1 teaspoon lemon zest
- Juice from 1 lemon
- ½ cup almond flour
- 4 boneless and skinless chicken breasts, 4 oz. each and cut in half
- 1 chopped scallion
- 2 tablespoons mustard
- 1 tablespoons olive oil
- 2 teaspoons tarragon

Directions:

1. In a shallow bowl, combine the lemon zest, almond flour, and pepper.

2. Wrap the chicken breast in plastic and pound them until they're ¼-inch thick.
3. Coat both sides of the chicken breasts with the almond mixture.
4. Pour the olive oil into a large skillet and set on medium heat.
5. Sear the chicken for about four minutes or until they're golden brown on each side. If you can't fit all the chicken in the pan at once, put the cooked chicken on a plate with tin foil over to keep it warm.
6. Once all the chicken is cooked and covered with foil, add the scallion to the pan and sauté for one minute.
7. Combine the mustard, tarragon, and lemon juice together. Mix well.
8. Divide the chicken onto plates, pour the sauce over it and season with salt and pepper before serving.

Chicken and Olives

Prep time: 10 minutes

Cook time: 15 minutes

Serving size: 4

Nutritional information: Calories-135; Carbs-12 grams; Fat-6 grams; Protein-10 grams

Ingredients:

- 4 boneless and skinless chicken breasts
- Juice from 1 lemon
- 2 tablespoons olive oil
- ¼ cup pitted and sliced green olives
- ½ cup sodium-free chicken stock
- 1 cup diced onion
- 1 ½ cups cubed tomatoes
- 1 tablespoon dried oregano
- 2 tablespoons minced garlic

Directions:

1. Pour the olive oil into a pan over medium heat.
2. Sauté the garlic for a couple of minutes.
3. Add the chicken and brown on both sides, should take about two minutes.
4. Combine the rest of the ingredients. Mix until fully incorporated.
5. Turn the heat down to simmer and cook for 13 minutes before serving.

Rosemary Baked Chicken Drumstick

Prep time: 5 minutes

Cook time: 1 hour

Serving size: 6

Nutritional information: Calories-163; Carbs-2 grams; Fat-6 grams; Protein-26 grams

Ingredients:

- 12 chicken drumsticks
- 1 teaspoon garlic powder
- 2 tablespoons chopped rosemary leaves (fresh is best)
- zest from 1 lemon
- Sea salt and ground black pepper to your desired taste

Directions:

1. Set the temperature of your oven to 350°F
2. Mix the ingredients minus the drumsticks in a small bowl.
3. Grease a 9 x 13-inch pan or line with parchment paper.
4. Layer the drumsticks in the pan and then rub the rosemary mixture on each side.
5. Place in the oven for one hour.

Moussaka

Prep time: 10 minutes

Cook time: 45 minutes

Serving size: 8

Nutritional information: Calories-338; Carbs-16 grams; Fat-20 grams; Protein-28 grams

Ingredients:

- 1 beaten egg
- 1 teaspoons dried oregano
- 1 cup unsweetened nonfat plain Greek yogurt
- 2 tablespoons Worcestershire sauce
- ½ teaspoon ground cinnamon
- ¼ teaspoon ground nutmeg
- ¼ cup grated parmesan cheese
- 2 tablespoon chopped parsley leaves
- 1 chopped onion
- 5 tablespoon olive oil, divided
- 1 sliced eggplant, not peeled
- 2 tablespoons tomato
- 1 pound ground turkey
- 14 oz. chopped tomatoes
- 1 seeded and chopped green bell pepper
- 3 minced garlic cloves
- 1 tablespoon Italian seasoning

Directions:

1. Preheat your oven to 400°F
2. Pour 3 tablespoons of olive oil into a large skillet to heat up on medium.
3. Brown the eggplant slices for three minutes on each side. Place on a paper towel to dry.

4. Pour the rest of the olive oil into the pan and combine the bell pepper and onion. Cook for five minutes then remove from the pan and set aside.
5. Set the turkey into the skillet and crumble while cooking for five minutes.
6. Add the garlic, tomatoes, oregano, cinnamon, and Italian seasoning. Stir and then combine the onion mixture. Stir and cook for five minutes.
7. Combine the egg, nutmeg, cheese, and yogurt into a small bowl.
8. Grease a baking pan and spread half of the meat mixture on the bottom.
9. Layer with the half of the eggplant and then add the rest of the meat before adding the remaining eggplant.
10. Spread the yogurt mixture on top.
11. Set in the oven and turn your timer to 20 minutes.
12. Sprinkle with parsley before serving.

Chicken Wrap

Prep time: 10 minutes

Cook time: none

Serving size: 2

Nutritional information: Calories-190; Carbs-15 grams; Fat-7 grams; Protein-7 grams

Ingredients:

- 1 sliced onion
- 2 tablespoons chopped roasted red peppers
- 6 skinless and boneless chicken breasts, cooked and shredded
- 2 whole wheat tortilla flatbread
- 4 tomato slices
- 2 slices of provolone cheese, can substitute for your favorite cheese
- 10 pitted and sliced kalamata olives
- Baby spinach

Directions:

1. Set the tortillas on a flat working surface.
2. Add the ingredients onto the flatbread starting with the chicken breasts, then cheese, and the toppings.
3. Roll them up and serve.

Mediterranean Pork Chops

Prep time: 10 minutes plus 30 minutes marinating

Cook time: 35 minutes

Serving size: 4

Nutritional information: Calories-368; Carbs-1 gram; Fat-28 grams; Protein-26 grams

Ingredients:

- 4 pork loin chops, 4 oz. each
- 1 tablespoon minced garlic
- 1 teaspoon chopped oregano
- 1 teaspoon chopped rosemary
- Sea salt and ground black pepper to taste

Directions:

1. Season the pork chops with salt and pepper on both sides.
2. Combine the rosemary, garlic, and oregano in a small bowl.
3. Rub the garlic paste on each side of the pork chops and let them marinate for 30 minutes at room temperature.
4. Preheat your oven to 350°F
5. Grease a baking pan with cooking oil or line a piece of parchment paper on the pan.
6. Set the chops on the baking sheet and in the oven for 35 minutes.

Marinara Meatballs

Prep time: 25 minutes

Cook time: 1 hour

Serving size: 8

Nutritional information: Calories-284; Carbs-10 grams; Fat-13 grams; Protein-32 grams

Ingredients for the sauce:

- 1 chopped onion
- 8 large tomatoes, peeled and cut into chunks
- 1 tablespoon minced garlic
- 1 cup low-sodium chicken broth
- 2 tablespoons olive oil
- 1 tablespoon chopped oregano
- 1 tablespoon chopped basil
- 2 tablespoons balsamic vinegar
- 1 bay leaf
- ¼ teaspoon red pepper flakes
- ¼ teaspoon ground black pepper
- ¼ teaspoon sea salt

Ingredients for the meatballs:

- 1 pound lean ground pork
- ¼ teaspoon ground black pepper
- 1 pound lean ground beef
- ¼ teaspoon sea salt
- 1 egg
- 1 cup almond flour
- 1 teaspoon minced garlic
- 1 teaspoon chopped oregano
- 1 teaspoon chopped parsley

Directions for the sauce:

1. Set a large saucepan over medium heat and pour in the olive oil.
2. Sauté the garlic and onions for two to three minutes.
3. Stir in the rest of the ingredients. Mix until fully incorporated.
4. Bring the sauce to a boil and then simmer for 30 minutes or until meatballs are cooked through.

Directions for the meatballs:

1. With the sauce simmering, combine all of the ingredients and stir well.
2. Roll the mixture into 1-inch balls.
3. Carefully drop them into the sauce and cook.
4. Remove the bay leaf and serve.

Turkey and Bean Chili

Prep time: 15 minutes

Cook time: 55 minutes

Serving size: 5

Nutritional information: Calories-377; Carbs-41 grams; Fat-7 grams; Protein-43 grams

Ingredients:

- 1 pound lean ground turkey breast
- 1 teaspoon olive oil
- 1 finely chopped jalapeno pepper
- 1 chopped onion
- 2 teaspoons ground cumin
- ¼ cup chili powder
- 2 teaspoons minced garlic
- 4 chopped tomatoes
- 1 cup rinsed and drained kidney beans
- 1 cup rinsed and drained chickpeas
- 1 cup rinsed and drained black beans
- Pinch of cayenne pepper

Directions:

1. Pour the oil into a large stockpot and turn the heat to medium.
2. Sauté the turkey for six to seven minutes or until it's fully cooked.
3. Combine the jalapeno pepper, onion, and garlic. Stir well and sauté for another four minutes.
4. Add the cayenne, tomatoes, cumin, chili powder, kidney beans, black beans, and chickpeas. Stir well.
5. Bring the chili to a boil and reduce to low heat. Simmer to 45 minutes and then serve.

Turkey with Peaches and Walnuts

Prep time: 10 minutes

Cook time: 1 hour

Serving size: 4

Nutritional information: Calories-500; Carbs-15 grams; Fat-14 grams; Protein-10 grams

Ingredients:

- 4 pitted peaches, cut into quarters
- 2 skinless, boneless, and sliced turkey breasts
- 1 chopped onion
- 1 tablespoon chopped cilantro
- 1 tablespoon chopped walnuts
- ¼ cup sodium-free chicken stock
- 2 tablespoons olive oil

Directions:

1. Preheat your oven to 390°F
2. Grease a roasting pan with oil.
3. Add in all of the ingredients except the cilantro. Mix well.
4. Place in the oven for one hour.
5. Sprinkle with cilantro before serving.

Sage Turkey Mix

Prep time: 10 minutes

Cook time: 40 minutes

Serving size: 4

Nutritional information: Calories-382; Carbs-17 grams; Fat-13 grams; Protein-33 grams

Ingredients:

- 1 cup sodium-free chicken stock
- 1 skinless and boneless turkey breast, cut into rough cubes
- 2 tablespoons avocado oil
- 2 tablespoons chopped sage
- 1 chopped onion
- 1 minced garlic clove

Directions:

1. Pour the avocado oil into a pan over medium-high heat.
2. Add the turkey and brown on each side for three minutes.
3. Combine the rest of the ingredients, toss, and reduce the heat to medium-low. Let it cook for 35 minutes.
4. Divide the mixture on plates and serve.

Turkey Burgers with Mango Salsa

Prep time: 15 minutes

Cook time: 10 minutes

Serving size: 6

Nutritional information: Calories-384; Carbs-27 grams; Fat-16 grams; Protein-34 grams

Ingredients:

- 1 ½ pounds ground turkey breast
- 2 peeled, pitted, and cubed mangos
- ½ minced jalapeno pepper
- 2 tablespoons olive oil
- ½ chopped onion
- 2 tablespoons chopped cilantro leaves
- 1 minced garlic clove
- Juice from 1 lime

Directions:

1. Divide the ground turkey into four patties.
2. Pour the olive oil into a large skillet over medium-high heat.
3. Layer the turkey burgers and cook each side for five minutes.
4. In a bowl, combine the rest of the ingredients to make the salsa. Mix well.

5. Spoon a little salsa over the turkey burgers before serving.

Pork Fajita Roll-Ups

Prep time: 10 minutes plus 1 hour marinating time

Cook time: 25 minutes

Serving size: 4

Nutritional information: Calories-293; Carbs-6 grams; Fat-17 grams; Protein-22 grams

Ingredients:

- 4 pork chops, 4 oz. each
- 1 tablespoon olive oil
- 1 teaspoon minced garlic
- 1 sliced yellow bell pepper
- 1 sliced red bell pepper
- ½ teaspoon ground cumin
- 1 teaspoon dried oregano
- 1 thinly sliced onion
- Zest and juice from 1 lime

Directions:

1. Whisk the lime juice, lime zest, olive oil, cumin, garlic, and oregano into a medium bowl.

2. On a flat surface, cut the pork chops horizontally through the middle, within a ½-inch cutting all the way through.
3. Spread the pork open and pound them until they're ¼-inch thick.
4. Set them in the bowl, cover, and marinate for one hour.
5. Turn your oven to 400°F
6. Take the pork chops out of the bowl and open them up again.
7. Add the onion and bell pepper slices to the chops and roll them up.
8. Secure the pork with toothpicks and set them seam-side down on a baking sheet.
9. Place in the oven for 25 minutes or until the pork is done.

Baked Parsley Lamb

Prep time: 10 minutes

Cook time: 15 minutes

Serving size: 4

Nutritional information: Calories-353; Carbs-0 grams; Fat-25 grams; Protein-26 grams

Ingredients:

- ¼ cup parsley sprigs
- 2 tablespoons olive oil, divided
- 1 tablespoon chopped thyme leaves
- 4 lamb chops, 5 oz. each
- 1 teaspoon minced garlic

Directions:

1. Preheat your oven to 400°F
2. Add 4 teaspoons olive oil, parsley, garlic, and thyme into a blender. Pulse until it forms a thick paste.
3. Pour the remaining olive oil into a large skillet set to medium-high heat.
4. Set the lamb chops in the skillet and sear the sides for about five minutes total.
5. Transfer the meat into a baking dish and spread the parsley mixture over them.
6. Set the chops into the oven for about 10 minutes or until they've reached your desired done-ness.

Fish and Seafood

Fish and Orzo

Prep time: 10 minutes

Cook time: 35 minutes

Serving size: 4

Nutritional information: Calories-402; Carbs-21 grams; Fat-21 grams; Protein-31 grams

Ingredients:

- Zest from 1 lemon
- 1 teaspoon crushed red pepper
- 2 chopped shallots
- 1 teaspoon minced garlic
- 1 teaspoon anchovy paste
- 1 tablespoon olive oil
- 2 tablespoon pitted and chopped black olives
- 1 tablespoon dried oregano
- 15 oz. crushed tomatoes
- 2 tablespoons drained capers
- 4 boneless cod fillets
- 3 cups sodium-free chicken stock
- 1 oz. crumbled feta cheese

- 1 tablespoon chopped parsley
- 1 cup orzo pasta

Directions:

1. Turn your oven to 375°F
2. Set an oven-safe pan on medium heat and pour in the olive oil.
3. Sauté the garlic, shallots, and red pepper for five minutes.
4. Combine the anchovy paste, black olives, oregano, capers, and tomatoes. Cook for five minutes.
5. Lay the fish on top and sprinkle with cheese and parsley.
6. Put the pan into the oven for 15 minutes.
7. While the fish is baking, set a pot to medium heat and pour in the chicken stock.
8. Add the orzo and lemon zest. Cook until it starts to boil and then reduce heat to simmer for 10 minutes.
9. Divide the orzo onto plates, add a fish on top and pour juices over for extra taste before serving.

Fish Cakes

Prep time: 10 minutes

Cook time: 10 minutes

Serving size: 6

Nutritional information: Calories-288; Carbs-22 grams; Fat-12 grams; Protein-7 grams

Ingredients:

- 1 chopped yellow onion
- 1 whisked egg
- 5 tablespoons olive oil
- 2 tablespoons chopped dill
- 20 oz. sardines, drained and mashed
- 1 minced garlic cloves
- 1 cup breadcrumbs
- 2 tablespoons lemon juice

Directions:

1. Combine all the ingredients together except the oil in a bowl. Mix until fully incorporated.
2. Shape the mixture into medium cakes.
3. Pour the oil into a pan and place on medium heat.
4. Layer the cakes in the pan and cook for five minutes per side.
5. Serve the cakes with your favorite salad.

Shrimp and Bean Salad

Prep time: 10 minutes

Cook time: 4 minutes

Serving size: 4

Nutritional information: Calories-207; Carbs-15 grams; Fat-13 grams; Protein-9 grams

Ingredients:

- 2 tablespoons olive oil
- ½ cup chopped red onion
- 1 pound peeled and deveined shrimp
- 4 handfuls of baby arugula
- 1 cup halved cherry tomatoes
- 30 oz. cannellini beans, drained and rinsed
- 1 tablespoon lemon zest

Ingredients for the dressing:

- Salt and pepper for seasoning
- ½ cup olive oil
- 2 minced garlic cloves
- 3 tablespoons of red wine vinegar

Directions:

1. Pour the olive oil into a skillet over medium-high heat.
2. Cook the shrimp for two minutes on each side.
3. In a bowl, combine all of the ingredients, excluding the ones for the dressing. Toss and set aside.
4. In a smaller bowl, whisk all of the ingredients for the dressing,
5. Pour the dressing over the salad, toss to mix, and enjoy.

Cod and Mushrooms

Prep time: 10 minutes

Cook time: 25 minutes

Serving size: 4

Nutritional information: Calories-257; Carbs-24 grams; Fat-10 grams; Protein-19 grams

Ingredients:

- 2 tablespoons balsamic vinegar
- 1 chopped red chili pepper
- 1 oz. crumbled feta cheese
- 1 tablespoon cilantro
- 2 boneless cod fillets
- 4 oz. sliced mushrooms
- 12 halved cherry tomatoes
- 1 pitted, peeled, and cubed avocado
- 4 tablespoons olive oil
- 8 oz. torn lettuce leaves
- Sea salt and black pepper to taste

Directions:

1. In a roasting pan, brush 2 tablespoons of oil on the cod. Sprinkle each side with salt and pepper. Set in the oven and broil for 15 minutes.

2. In a skillet, pour in the rest of the olive oil and heat up on medium.
3. Sauté the mushrooms for five minutes.
4. Toss in the rest of the ingredients and gently stir. Cook for another five minutes.
5. Divide the skillet mixture onto plates and set the cod on top before serving.

Creamy Curry Salmon

Prep time: 10 minutes

Cook time: 20 minutes

Serving size: 2

Nutritional information: Calories-284; Carbs-27 grams; Fat-14 grams; Protein-31 grams

Ingredients:

- ½ teaspoon chopped mint
- 1 cup Greek yogurt
- 2 boneless and cubed salmon fillets
- 1 tablespoon olive oil
- 2 teaspoons curry powder
- 1 tablespoon chopped basil
- 1 minced garlic clove

Directions:

1. Pour olive oil into a skillet and set to medium heat.
2. Layer the salmon in the pan and cook for three minutes or until it's heated through.
3. Combine the rest of the ingredients and mix well. Cook for another 15 minutes.
4. Season with sea salt and pepper before serving.

Trout with Tzatziki Sauce

Prep time: 10 minutes

Cook time: 10 minutes

Serving size: 4

Nutritional information: Calories-393; Carbs-18 grams; Fat-18 grams; Protein-39 grams

Ingredients:

- 1 ½ teaspoon ground coriander
- Juice from ½ lime
- 4 boneless trout fillets
- 2 tablespoons avocado oil
- 1 teaspoon minced garlic
- 1 teaspoon sweet paprika

Ingredients for the sauce:

- 4 minced garlic cloves
- 1 chopped cucumber
- 1 teaspoon white vinegar
- 1 ½ cup Greek yogurt
- 1 tablespoon olive oil

Directions:

1. Set a pan to medium-high heat and add the avocado oil.
2. In a small bowl, combine the lime juice, coriander, garlic, and paprika. Rub on both sides of the fish.
3. Cook the trout until both sides are a golden brown, about four minutes.
4. In a separate bowl, mix the ingredients for the sauce together.
5. Pour the sauce over the trout once it's on a plate and serve.

Shrimp Mojo de Ajo

Prep time: 10 minutes

Cook time: 40 minutes

Serving size: 4

Nutritional information: Calories-354; Carbs-24 grams; Fat-15 grams; Protein-30 grams

Ingredients:

- 5 minced garlic cloves
- 8 oz. quartered mushrooms
- ¼ cup olive oil
- ⅛ teaspoon cayenne pepper, more if you like
- 1 pound peeled and deveined shrimp with tails removed
- 2 cups cooked brown rice
- Juice from 1 lime
- ¼ teaspoon sea salt
- ¼ cup chopped cilantro leaves

Directions:

1. Set a saucepan over low heat.
2. Combine the garlic, olive oil, and cayenne. Cook until it comes to low simmer, just when bubbles are starting to come to the surface.
3. Turn the heat down to simmer. Cook for 30 minutes and stir occasionally.
4. Strain the garlic from the oil and set aside.
5. Pour the oil into a large skillet over medium heat. Allow the oil to come to a shimmer.
6. Toss in the mushrooms and cook for five minutes.
7. Combine the shrimp, sea salt, and lime juice. Continue to cook for four more minutes or until the shrimp is pink.

8. Stir in the cilantro and garlic.
9. Divide the rice onto place, pour the mixture on top, and serve.

Five-Spice Calamari

Prep time: 15 minutes and 1 hour to marinate

Cook time: 10 minutes

Serving size: 4

Nutritional information: Calories-148; Carbs-7 grams; Fat-5 grams; Protein-18 grams

Ingredients:

- 1 tablespoon olive oil
- 1 teaspoon five-spice powder
- 1 minced red bell pepper
- Zest from 1 lime
- 4 large squid
- 2 tablespoons chopped cilantro

Directions:

1. Clean and split the squid open, so you can cut the tentacles into small pieces (calamari).
2. Combine the olive oil and five-spice powder in a medium bowl.

3. Stir in the calamari and marinade in the fridge for one hour.
4. Set your oven to broil.
5. Lay a piece of parchment paper or grease a baking pan.
6. Layer the calamari on the baking pan and set in the oven for ten minutes. Turnover at the five minute mark.
7. Set the calamari on a plate and garnish with lime zest, cilantro (if you want more), and red pepper before serving.

Vegetable Baked Salmon

Prep time: 15 minutes

Cook time: 20 minutes

Serving size: 4

Nutritional information: Calories-232; Carbs-12 grams; Fat-6 grams; Protein-36 grams

Ingredients:

- 2 cups cherry tomatoes
- 2 tablespoons minced garlic
- 5 quartered and cleaned bok choy
- Juice from 1 lemon
- 1 thinly sliced onion

- 4 salmon fillets, rinsed and patted dry, 6 oz. each

Directions:

1. Turn your oven to 400°F
2. Tear off two large sheets of foil and place them on the baking sheet, making sure they overlap in the middle.
3. Combine the bok choy, onion, lemon juice, cherry tomatoes, and garlic in a large bowl. Mix well.
4. Arrange the vegetables along the middle of the foil.
5. Layer the salmon on top of the vegetables.
6. Tear off a third piece of foil and place that on top of the fish. Crimp the edges of the foil together so you create a packet.
7. Set in the oven and turn your time for 20 minutes.
8. Sprinkle the salmon with sea salt and pepper to your taste bud's desire before enjoying.

Sun-Dried Tomato Cod

Prep time: 10 minutes

Cook time: 20 minutes

Serving size: 4

Nutritional information: Calories-239; Carbs-11 grams; Fat-9 grams; Protein-33 grams

Ingredients:

- 2 tablespoons dried basil
- 2 tablespoons olive oil
- 15 oz. sodium-free diced tomatoes
- ½ cup chopped sun-dried tomatoes
- 2 teaspoons minced garlic
- 1 sliced onion
- 4 cod fillets, 6 oz. each
- Pinch of red pepper flakes

Directions:

1. Turn your oven to 400°F
2. Pour the olive oil into an oven-safe skillet over medium heat.
3. Sauté the garlic and onions until they're soft.
4. Add in the sun-dried tomatoes, basil, tomatoes, and red pepper flakes.
5. Slide the sauce to the side of the skillet and layer the cod.
6. Scoop the sauce over the cod and then place in the oven.
7. Bake for 15 to 17 minutes or until the fish flakes easily.
8. Sprinkle with sea salt and pepper for seasoning.

Honey Salmon

Prep time: 10 minutes

Cook time: 20 minutes

Serving size: 4

Nutritional information: Calories-300; Carbs-11 grams; Fat-18 grams; Protein-24 grams

Ingredients:

- 4 salmon fillets, 6 oz and patted dry
- 2 tablespoons raw honey
- 1 tablespoon olive oil
- 2 tablespoons sesame seeds
- 4 cups chopped collard greens

Directions:

1. Preheat your oven to 400°F
2. Place a piece of parchment paper on a baking sheet.
3. Line the fish on the paper.
4. Brush honey on top of the fish.
5. Sprinkle with sesame seeds.
6. Place in the oven for 20 minutes or until it's cooked through.
7. When the fish is baking, pour the olive oil into a large skillet over medium heat.

8. Sauté the collard greens for 10 minutes.
9. Season the greens with salt and pepper.
10. Divide the fish onto plates and top with collard greens before serving.

Trout with Lemon Sauce

Prep time: 10 minutes

Cook time: 20 minutes

Serving size: 4

Nutritional information: Calories-295; Carbs-9 grams; Fat-12 grams; Protein-35 grams

Ingredients:

- 4 trout fillets, 6 oz. each
- 1 tablespoon olive oil
- 1 tablespoon cornstarch
- 1 tablespoon lemon zest
- ¼ cup lemon juice, freshly squeezed
- 1 tablespoon raw honey
- ½ cup low-fat plain Greek yogurt
- 1 tablespoon chopped thyme
- 2 tablespoon chopped scallion greens

Directions:

1. Turn your oven to 400°F
2. Pour the olive oil into an oven-safe skillet. Set the temperature to medium high.
3. Sear the trout on both sides for about 6 minutes.
4. Set the pan into the oven for 15 minutes.
5. While the fish is baking, make the sauce by placing a small saucepan over medium-high heat.
6. Combine the cornstarch, lemon juice, lemon zest, thyme, and hone. Whisk together and cook for three minutes. The sauce should thicken.
7. Turn off the heat and add in the yogurt. Whisk well.
8. Top the fish with the sauce. Sprinkle on the scallions before serving.

Salmon Wrap

Prep time: 10 minutes

Cook time: 15 minutes

Serving size: 4

Nutritional information: Calories-377; Carbs-19 grams; Fat-23 grams; Protein-26 grams

Ingredients:

- 1 medium diced apple
- 1 tablespoon olive oil
- 1 head of romaine lettuce
- 1 tablespoon chopped mint, fresh
- 1 pound salmon fillet
- 2 limes
- 1 diced avocado
- 1 diced tomato

Directions:

1. Preheat your oven to 425°F
2. Place a piece of aluminum foil on top of a baking sheet.
3. Add the salmon on the foil.
4. Season it with salt and pepper to your taste.
5. Slice one lime and then spread evenly on top of the fish.
6. Place in the oven for 15 minutes.
7. While the fish is baking, combine the avocado, apple, and tomato into a medium bowl. Toss well.
8. In a separate bowl, whisk the olive oil, juice from the other lime, and mint.
9. Wash and dry the lettuce leaves.
10. When the salmon is done, flake it into the apple mixture.
11. Pour the oil mixture on top. Mix until ingredients are fully incorporated.
12. Lay the lettuce leaves on a flat surface.
13. Scoop ¼ of the mixture into the center of each leaf.
14. Roll up before serving.

Haddock Asian-Style

Prep time: 10 minutes

Cook time: 15 minutes

Serving size: 4

Nutritional information: Calories-194; Carbs-6 grams; Fat-3 grams; Protein-34 grams

Ingredients:

- 4 haddock fillets, 6 oz. each
- 1 cup oyster mushrooms
- 1 cup finely shredded green cabbage
- 4 baby bok choy, trim ends
- 1 thinly sliced red bell pepper
- 1 ½ teaspoon rice vinegar
- 2 teaspoons peeled and grated ginger
- 3 onions, thinly sliced diagonally
- 2 tablespoons liquid aminos
- 1 ½ teaspoons sesame oil

Directions:

1. Preheat your oven to 400°F
2. Cut eight 15-inch squares of parchment paper. Arrange two squares each on two baking pans.

3. Divide the mushrooms, bok choy, bell pepper, and cabbage evenly among the four parchment pieces.
4. Set a haddock on top of each.
5. Top with green onions.
6. Whisk together the aminos, oil, ginger, and vinegar in a small bowl. Scoop the mixture evenly over the fish.
7. Take the remaining squares of parchment paper and place on top of each fish. Fold the edges to create a seal.
8. Set in the oven for 15 minutes or until you can flake the fish with a fork.
9. Transfer each packet onto a plate for serving.

Fish Tacos

Prep time: 20 minutes plus 15 minutes to marinate

Cook time: 11 minutes

Serving size: 4

Nutritional information: Calories-290; Carbs-28 grams; Fat-8 grams; Protein-27 grams

Ingredients for the white sauce:

- ½ teaspoon ground cumin
- ½ teaspoon dill
- ½ cup nonfat plain Greek yogurt
- ½ teaspoon crushed oregano

- Juice from 1 lime
- 1 teaspoon sriracha hot sauce

Ingredients for the tacos:

- 4 tablespoons olive oil, plus a bit more for grill
- ½ teaspoon oregano
- ½ head of red cabbage, thinly sliced and cored
- ½ thinly sliced onion
- ½ cup thinly sliced radishes
- 8 organic corn tortillas, 6 inches each
- ½ cup chopped cilantro
- 1 pound white fish, such as cod or catfish
- 1 minced garlic clove
- 2 halved limes
- ¼ teaspoon chili powder
- 1 teaspoon ground cumin

Directions for the tacos:

1. Set the fish in a baking dish and squeeze lime over it.
2. Sprinkle the fish with chili powder, cumin, oregano, garlic, and three teaspoons of olive oil.
3. Evenly coat the fish with the marinate. Set in the fridge for 15 minutes.
4. Combine the onion, radishes, cilantro, and juice from another lime in a medium bowl.
5. Pour in the rest of the olive oil and toss to combine.

Directions for the white sauce:

1. Combine all of the white sauce ingredients into a small bowl. Whisk until it's fully incorporated.

To assemble the tacos:

1. Take one tortilla at the time, warm both sides up in a medium skillet over medium-high heat.
2. Using a clean dishcloth, keep the tortillas warm by wrapping them and set aside.
3. Using an outdoor grill or a grill pan, brush the grates.
4. Place the grill pan over medium-high heat and let it warm up.
5. Take the fish out of the marinade and set each piece on the grill.
6. Cook the fish for about three minutes and then flip it. Cook for another three minutes.
7. Transfer the fish onto a plate.
8. Flake some of the fish off and place it in a tortilla.
9. Top it with the radish mixture.
10. Drizzle the white sauce on the tacos before serving.

Nut-Breaded Cod with Lemon

Prep time: 15 minutes

Cook time: 10 minutes

Serving size: 4

Nutritional information: Calories-417; Carbs-6 grams; Fat-20 grams; Protein-52 grams

Ingredients:

- 1 tablespoon lemon zest
- 4 cod fillets, 6 oz. each
- 2 whisked eggs
- 1 cup slivered almonds
- ½ teaspoon chopped thyme

Directions:

1. Preheat your oven to 450°F
2. Place a piece of aluminum foil on top of a baking sheet
3. In a blender, mix the lemon zest, almonds, and thyme. Pulse until the texture is coarsely ground.
4. Transfer the mixture onto a plate.
5. Use a paper towel to pat the fish dry.
6. In a shallow bowl, pour the eggs.
7. Dip the fish into the egg mixture and then the almond mixture.
8. Make sure it is fully coated and then place on the baking sheet.
9. Repeat the process with the rest of the fish.
10. Lightly spray the breaded fish with olive oil.
11. Set in the oven for 10 minutes or until the fish begins to flake.

Salmon with Pistachio Crust

Prep time: 15 minutes

Cook time: 15 minutes

Serving size: 4

Nutritional information: Calories-368; Carbs-6 grams; Fat-22 grams; Protein-39 grams

Ingredients:

- 2 tablespoons water
- 1 egg
- ½ cup ground almonds
- 4 salmon fillets, 6 oz. each
- ½ cup finely chopped pistachios
- ½ teaspoon chopped thyme

Directions:

1. Preheat your oven to 450°F
2. Line a baking sheet with aluminum foil
3. Whisk the egg and water in a small bowl.
4. In a separate bowl, combine the almonds, thyme, and pistachios.
5. Using paper towels, pat the fish dry.
6. Dip the fish into the egg and then the pistachios mixture.

7. Place the fillet onto the foil and repeat with the rest of the fish.
8. Set it in the oven and turn your timer to 15 minutes.

Drinks and Dessert

Strawberry Lemonade

Prep time: 5 minutes, plus 2 hours to chill

Cook time: none

Serving size: 2

Nutritional information: Calories-77; Carbs-16 grams; Fat-1 gram; Protein-1 gram

Ingredients:

- ¾ cup lemon juice, freshly squeezed
- ¼ cup lime juice, freshly squeezed
- 1 cup sliced strawberries
- 2 cups water
- 1 tablespoon honey
- 4 ice cubes

Directions:

1. In a pitcher or a nonreactive bowl, combine the lime juice, honey, lemon juice, and water. Stir until well blended.
2. Crush the strawberries with the back of the spoon. Stir them into the lemonade.
3. Refrigerate the drink for 2 hours, so the liquid can infuse and chill.
4. Before enjoying, divide the ice cubes into two glasses and serve.

Iced Green Tea

Prep time: 10 minutes plus 2 hours to chill

Cook time: none

Serving size: 2

Nutritional information: Calories-11; Carbs-2 grams; Fat-0 grams; Protein-0 grams

Ingredients:

- 2 green tea bags
- 1 tablespoon chopped fresh mint
- 3 cups boiling water
- 2-inch fresh ginger, peeled and grated
- ½ teaspoon chopped thyme

- 6 ice cubes
- Garnish with fresh mint sprigs

Directions:

1. In a medium bowl, mix the ginger, thyme, boiling water, tea bags, and mint. Stir well and let it sit for five minutes.
2. Take the bags out but squeeze them to remove all of the liquid.
3. Using a fine-mesh sieve, pour the liquid into a container. Discard any solids in the sieve.
4. Refrigerate the tea for at least two hours.
5. Transfer the liquid into a blender and drop in the ice cubes. Mix until you have a smooth and thick texture.
6. Garnish with the mint sprigs before serving.

Green Apple Smoothie

Prep time: 10 minutes

Cook time: none

Serving size: 2

Nutritional information: Calories-286; Carbs-23 grams; Fat-22 grams; Protein-3 grams

Ingredients:

- 1 peeled, cored, and chopped green apple
- 1 cup unsweetened coconut milk
- 2 cups spinach leaves
- 1 peeled and pitted avocado
- 1 teaspoon chopped thyme, fresh is best
- 3 ice cubes

Directions:

1. Combine the coconut milk, apple, spinach, thyme, and avocado into a blender. Mix until smooth.
2. Add the ice cubes and blend until you have a thick and smooth smoothie to enjoy.

Coconut Custard

Prep time: 10 minutes

Cook time: 45 minutes

Serving size: 4

Nutritional information: Calories-146; Carbs-7 grams; Fat-10 grams; Protein-6 grams

Ingredients:

- 2 cups canned coconut milk
- 3 large eggs
- 2 teaspoons pure vanilla extract

- 1 tablespoon honey
- ¼ cup unsweetened shredded coconut
- ¼ teaspoon ground nutmeg
- A dash of sea salt

Directions:

1. Set the temperature of your oven to 350°F
2. Whisk the eggs, vanilla, honey, salt, and nutmeg in a medium bowl. Ensure it's well blended.
3. Place a small saucepan on medium heat and pour in the coconut milk.
4. Allow the milk to simmer before removing it from heat to whisk in the egg mixture.
5. Using a fine-mesh sieve, pour the mixture into an 8 x 8-inch baking dish.
6. Set this dish into a large baking dish and pour the hot water into the larger dish. The water should come halfway up to the custard pan. Do your best not to spill any water into the mixture so you don't ruin its consistency.
7. Set in the oven for about 45 to 50 minutes or until a knife or toothpick inserted into the center of the custard comes out clean.
8. Place the custard pan on a wire rack for an hour to cool.
9. Refrigerate the custard.
10. Sprinkle the shredded coconut over it before serving.

Dark Chocolate Chia Pudding

Prep time: 15 minutes plus 2 hours to thicken

Cook time: 5 minutes

Serving size: 4

Nutritional information: Calories-125; Carbs-19 grams; Fat-8 grams; Protein-5 grams

Ingredients:

- ¼ cup unsweetened cocoa powder
- ½ chop chia seeds
- 2 cups unsweetened almond milk
- 2 tablespoons honey
- 1 teaspoon pure vanilla extract
- Garnish with strawberries (optional)

Directions:

1. Place a small saucepan over low heat.
2. Combine the vanilla, almond milk, honey, and cocoa powder. Mix well.
3. Let the mixture heat until the cocoa powder is completely dissolved, about four minutes.
4. Pour into a medium bowl.
5. Add in the chia seeds and mix.
6. Place the bowl into the fridge for 2 hours but stir the pudding every ½ hour.

7. Once the pudding is thick, garnish with strawberries if you desire and enjoy.

Lemon and Blueberry Curd

Prep time: 10 minutes plus chilling time

Cook time: 5 minutes

Serving size: 4

Nutritional information: Calories-249; Carbs-20 grams; Fat-18 grams; Protein-3 grams

Ingredients:

- 2 tablespoons raw honey
- Juice and zest from 1 lemon
- 2 cups blueberries
- 4 eggs yolks
- ¼ cup melted coconut oil
- 1 teaspoon pure vanilla extract

Directions:

1. Place a medium saucepan over medium heat.
2. Combine the honey, egg yolks, coconut oil, lemon juice, lemon zest, and vanilla. Whisk the mixture constantly for five minutes, or until it thickens.
3. Pour the curd through a sieve and into a bowl.

4. Cover the curd by pressing plastic wrap down to its surface.
5. Set in the refrigerator until it's cold.
6. Divide the blueberries and scoop the curd on top before enjoying.

Baked Walnut Pears

Prep time: 15 minutes

Cook time: 20 minutes

Serving size: 4

Nutritional information: Calories-360; Carbs-33 grams; Fat-22 grams; Protein-7 grams

Ingredients:

- 1 cup chopped walnuts
- 4 cored pears, leave whole
- 2 tablespoons almond butter
- ¼ cup dried cherries
- 2 tablespoons rolled oats
- ¼ teaspoon ground cinnamon

Directions:

1. Set your oven to 400°F
2. In an 8 x 8-inch baking dish, stand the pears

3. Combine the rest of the ingredients into a small bowl. Mix until it's fully incorporated.
4. Scoop the filling into the center of the pears.
5. Add them into the oven for about 20 minutes or until they're tender.

Sauce and Dressing

Spicy Almond Dressing

Prep time: 5 to 10 minutes

Cook time: none

Serving size: 1 cup

Nutritional information: calories-98; carbs-3 grams; fat-9 grams; protein-3 grams

Ingredients:

- ⅔ cups water
- 3 tablespoons almond butter
- 2 teaspoons curry powder
- Salt and pepper for seasoning

Directions:

1. In a bowl, add the almond butter and then one tablespoon of water. Stir the mixture before you add another tablespoon of water. Repeat this process until all the water is thoroughly mixed with the butter.
2. Combine the rest of the ingredients and stir well. Taste and add any more seasoning you feel necessary.
3. Pour the dressing into an airtight container and store in the fridge for 7 to 10 days.

Turmeric Tahini Dressing

Prep time: 5 to 10 minutes

Cook time: none

Serving size: 1 cup

Nutritional information: calories-208; carbs-3 grams; fat-21 grams; protein-3 grams

Ingredients:

- 3 tablespoons olive oil
- 3 tablespoons tahini
- 1 teaspoons turmeric powder
- ⅔ cup water
- Pinch of salt and pepper

Directions:

1. In a bowl pour in the olive oil and tahini. Combine well.
2. Mix the turmeric into the bowl.
3. Add in the water one tablespoon at a time, stirring the ingredients until they are fully incorporated before adding another tablespoon of water. Repeat this process until all of the water is mixed into the bowl.
4. Season the dressing to your taste.
5. Pour into an airtight container and store it for up to a week in your fridge.

Smoked Paprika Dressing

Prep time: 5 to 10 minutes

Cook time: none

Serving size: 1 cup

Nutritional information: calories-291; carbs-14 grams; fat-25 grams; protein-6 grams

Ingredients:

- Juice from ½ of a lemon
- 3 tablespoons cashew butter
- ⅔ cup water
- 2 teaspoons smoked paprika powder

- Salt for seasoning

Directions:

1. Pour the lemon juice into a bowl and stir in the cashew butter.
2. Add one tablespoon of water at a time, ensuring the ingredients are well mixed before adding in the next tablespoon. Repeat this process until all the water is incorporated and you have the consistency you desire.
3. Combine the paprika powder and salt. Adjust seasonings to your taste.
4. Transfer the dressing into an airtight container. It can sit in the fridge for up to 7 days.

Sesame Orange Sauce for Stir-Fry

Prep time: 5 minutes

Cook time: none

Serving size: 1 cup

Nutritional information: Calories-48; Carbs-4 grams; Fat-3 grams; Protein-1 gram

Ingredients:

- ¼ cup low-sodium chicken broth
- 1 tablespoon sesame oil
- 2 tablespoons coconut aminos
- 1 tablespoon arrowroot powder
- 1 tablespoon sesame seeds
- 1 tablespoon orange zest
- ½ cup orange juice, freshly squeezed

Directions:

- Combine all the ingredients together in a bowl. Whisk well.
- Keep the sauce in an air-tight container for up to seven days in the refrigerator.

Fiery Peanut Sauce

Prep time: 10 minutes

Cook time: none

Serving size: 1 ½ cups

Nutritional information: Calories-83; Carbs-3 grams; Fat-7 grams; Protein-3 grams

Ingredients:

- ½ cup coconut milk
- 1 teaspoon minced garlic
- Juice and zest from 1 lime
- ½ cup natural peanut butter
- 2 teaspoons coconut aminos
- 1 teaspoons chopped cilantro leaves, fresh
- A dash of red pepper flakes

Directions:

1. Whisk together all of the ingredients in a small bowl. Ensure it's fully incorporated.
2. Store in a sealed container for up to seven days.

Tomato Dressing

Prep time: 15 minutes

Cook time: none

Serving size: 1 cup

Nutritional information: Calories-130; Carbs-2 grams; Fat-0 grams; Protein-14 grams

Ingredients:

- 1 tablespoon minced basil leaves

- ½ cup olive oil
- 6 sun-dried tomatoes
- 2 tablespoons minced garlic
- 3 tablespoons balsamic vinegar
- Season with sea salt and black pepper

Directions:

1. Combine the garlic, vinegar, tomatoes, and basil in a blender. Pulse until smooth.
2. Transfer the mixture into a small bowl.
3. Add the olive oil and whisk well.
4. Season with pepper and salt to your desire.
5. Store in a sealed container for up to a week in the fridge.

Easy Marinara Sauce

Prep time: 10 minutes

Cook time: 25 minutes

Serving size: 4

Nutritional information: Calories-105; Carbs-10 grams; Fat-7 grams; Protein-2 grams

Ingredients:

- 2 tablespoons chopped oregano leaves
- 1 tablespoon chopped basil leaves
- 2 tablespoons olive oil
- 2 teaspoons minced garlic
- 4 cups diced tomatoes
- 1 chopped onion

Directions:

1. Pour the olive oil in a large saucepan over medium heat.
2. Sauté the garlic and onions until soft, about three minutes.
3. Combine the oregano, basil, and tomatoes.
4. Bring the sauce to a boil and reduce the heat to low. Simmer for 20 minutes.
5. Season the marinara with salt and pepper for seasoning.

Conclusion

One of the most important takeaways from this book is that PCOS is a manageable condition. It will take time to understand the syndrome and get used to following a healthy diet; it's not something that you can quickly learn from your doctor. You will find yourself doing your own research, and noticing that some of your symptoms might be different than those of other people you meet in support groups. You'll also realize that you react to some foods better than others. All of this is perfectly fine, and shouldn't worry you.

It's important that you take time to focus on yourself, so you don't become too anxious or depressed. I know that it's hard, especially when you're first diagnosed. You have so many questions, and sometimes you feel that your doctors can't even answer them. You might start to lose patience because you don't understand the condition, or what's happening to your body.

You will face a lot of frustrating and sad moments. There are a lot of challenges, but you need to do your best to manage your mood. Find strategies that work to help care for yourself, such as going for a walk, exercising, taking a hot bubble bath with epsom salt and candles. You can also use an essential oil diffuser to help in the self-care part of your life.

If you find yourself struggling, don't be afraid to reach out for help. Other than support groups on Facebook or through your friends and family, there are therapists. Ask your doctor to refer you to a counselor who can help you manage your mood.

Above all, remember that you are strong. You will learn how to manage PCOS. Your diagnosis doesn't determine your life.

References

Adams, R., & Brown, A. (2019). *PCOS diet: 2 books in 1 prediabetes & PCOS cookbook. learn to live a healthy, energetic lifestyle and discover how to reverse prediabetes and reduce insulin resistance to eliminating PCOS symptoms.* https://www.amazon.com/PCOS-Diet-Prediabetes-Resistance-Eliminating-ebook/dp/B082V3LB21?ie=UTF8&redirect=true&ref_=ku_mi_rw_edp

Allen, L. (2019, January 4). *Healthy breakfast smoothie.* Tastes Better From Scratch. https://tastesbetterfromscratch.com/healthy-breakfast-smoothie/

CDC. (2019, August 12). *PCOS (polycystic ovary syndrome) and diabetes.* Centers for Disease Control and Prevention. https://www.cdc.gov/diabetes/basics/pcos.html

Could insulin-resistance diet lower your diabetes risk? (n.d.). WebMD. Retrieved June 18, 2020, from https://www.webmd.com/diabetes/diabetes-insulin-resistance-diet#:~:text=You%20don

Fertility Answers. (2017, September 20). *9 PCOS diet tips*. Fertility Answers. https://www.fertilityanswers.com/9-pcos-diet-tips/

Galan, N. (2020a, January 17). *Learn about the relationship between PCOS and inflammation*. Verywell Health. https://www.verywellhealth.com/the-relationship-between-pcos-and-inflammation-2616649

Galan, N. (2020b, April 3). *How to know if you are ovulating with PCOS*. Verywell Health. https://www.verywellhealth.com/pcos-how-do-i-know-if-im-ovulating-regularly-2616460

Galan, N. (2020c, June 16). *Signs of insulin resistance*. Healthline. https://www.healthline.com/health/diabetes/insulin-resistance-symptoms#symptoms

Gunjan. (2017, December 13). *5 ingredient cranberry quinoa granola [vegan + GF]* kiipfit.com. Kiipfit.Com. https://kiipfit.com/5-ingredient-cranberry-quinoa-granola/#wprm-recipe-container-6090

Gunnars, K. (2018, July 24). *Mediterranean diet 101: A meal plan and beginner's guide*. Healthline. https://www.healthline.com/nutrition/mediterranean-diet-meal-plan#bottom-line

Harrar, S. (2017). *What causes PCOS? And how will it affect my body?* EndocrineWeb.

https://www.endocrineweb.com/conditions/polycystic-ovary-syndrome-pcos/what-causes-pcos-how-will-it-affect-body

Health Direct. (2019, December). *PCOS and pregnancy.* Pregnancybirthbaby.Org.Au; {{meta.dc.publisher}}. https://www.pregnancybirthbaby.org.au/pcos-and-pregnancy

Hitti, M. (2006, February). *How to use the glycemic index.* WebMD; WebMD. https://www.webmd.com/diabetes/guide/glycemic-index-good-versus-bad-carbs

Kelly, C. C. J., Lyall, H., Petrie, J. R., Gould, G. W., Connell, J. M. C., & Sattar, N. (2001). Low grade chronic inflammation in women with polycystic ovarian syndrome. The *Journal of Clinical Endocrinology & Metabolism, 86*(6), 2453–2455. https://doi.org/10.1210/jcem.86.6.7580

Link, L. (2018, March 22). *5 signs you have chronic inflammation and what to do about it.* Parsley Health. https://www.parsleyhealth.com/blog/5-signs-chronic-inflammation/

Link, R. (2020, June 2). *Glycemic index: What it is and how to use it.* Healthline. https://www.healthline.com/nutrition/glycemic-index#effects-of-cooking-ripening

McKittrick, M. (2019, August 22). *Newly diagnosed with PCOS? 14 tips to get you started.* Martha McKittrick Nutrition. https://www.marthamckittricknutrition.com/newly-diagnosed-with-pcos-14-tips-to-get-you-started/

Mira. (2016, May 28). *My PCOS kitchen - A simple keto breakfast.* My PCOS Kitchen. https://www.mypcoskitchen.com/keto-breakfast/#wprm-recipe-container-3898

Nature's Best. (n.d.). *PCOS and depression: How to manage your emotions.* Nature's Best. Retrieved June 14, 2020, from https://www.naturesbest.co.uk/pharmacy/polycystic-ovary-syndrome/pcos-and-depression-how-to-manage-your-emotions/

Poulton, T. (2014, July 24). *PCOS diet breakfast ideas.* PCOS Diet Support. https://www.pcosdietsupport.com/recipes/pcos-breakfast-ideas/

Reproductive Facts. (2014). *Polycystic ovary syndrome (PCOS).* Www.Reproductivefacts.Org. https://www.reproductivefacts.org/news-and-publications/patient-fact-sheets-and-booklets/documents/fact-sheets-and-info-booklets/polycystic-ovary-syndrome-pcos/

Sandler, L. (2019). *Mediterranean diet cookbook: 550 quick, easy and healthy mediterranean diet recipes for everyday cooking.* https://www.amazon.com/Mediterranean-Diet-Cookbook-Healthy-Everyday-ebook/dp/B07QR2KTQF?ie=UTF8&redirect=true&ref_=ku_mi_rw_edp

Shaw, M. (2015, November 25). *7 life changing tips to help you manage and alleviate PCOS.* Madeleine Shaw. https://madeleineshaw.com/7-life-changing-tips-to-help-you-manage-and-alleviate-pcos/

SitFlow. (n.d.). *8 ways to increase your daily physical activity.* SitFlow. Retrieved June 15, 2020, from https://sitflow.com/blogs/news/8-ways-to-increase-your-daily-physical-activity

Smith, M. (2019). *The mediterranean diet: Mediterranean diet for beginners, mediterranean diet plan, meal plan recipes, cookbook diet, mediterranean diet weight loss, burn fat and reset your metabolism.* https://www.amazon.com/MEDITERRANEAN-DIET-Mediterranean-mediterranean-metabolism-ebook/dp/B07QLJP58L?ie=UTF8&redirect=true&ref_=ku_mi_rw_edp

Spencer, T. (2017). *PCOS diet for the newly diagnosed: Your all-in-one guide to eliminating PCOS symptoms with the insulin resistance diet.* Rockridge Press. https://www.amazon.com/PCOS-Diet-Newly-

Diagnosed-All-ebook/dp/B071VCP545?ie=UTF8&redirect=true&ref_=ku_mi_rw_edp

Spencer, T. (2018). *The easy PCOS diet cookbook: Fuss-Free recipes for busy people on the insulin resistance diet.* Rockridge Press. https://www.amazon.com/Easy-PCOS-Diet-Cookbook-Resistance-ebook/dp/B07B8BSKBV?ie=UTF8&redirect=true&ref_=ku_mi_rw_edp

Spencer, T., & Koslo, J. (2016). *The insulin resistance diet plan & cookbook: Lose weight, manage PCOS, and prevent prediabetes.* Rockridge Press. https://www.amazon.com/Insulin-Resistance-Diet-Plan-Cookbook-ebook/dp/B01CVVP5M8?ie=UTF8&redirect=true&ref_=ku_mi_rw_edp

Spencer, T., & Koslo, J. (2017). *The insulin resistance diet for PCOS: A 4-week meal plan and cookbook to lose weight, boost fertility, and fight inflammation.* Rockridge Press. https://www.amazon.com/Insulin-Resistance-Diet-PCOS-Inflammation-ebook/dp/B01N4PSAEK?ie=UTF8&redirect=true&ref_=ku_mi_rw_edp

Spritzler, F. (2018, December 13). *Anti-Inflammatory diet 101: How to reduce inflammation naturally.* Healthline.

https://www.healthline.com/nutrition/anti-inflammatory-diet-101#other-tips

Watson, S. (2015, August 3). *Polycystic ovary syndrome (PCOS): Symptoms, causes, and treatment.* Healthline; Healthline Media. https://www.healthline.com/health/polycystic-ovary-disease#causes

Witkin, G. (2018, September 5). *PCOS: The mental, emotional, and physical.* Psychology Today. https://www.psychologytoday.com/us/blog/the-chronicles-infertility/201809/pcos-the-mental-emotional-and-physical

Printed in Great Britain
by Amazon